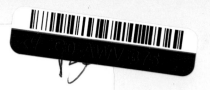

THE MEDICATED SOCIETY

THE
MEDICATED
SOCIETY

EDITED BY Samuel Proger, M.D.

*Sponsored by the Lowell Institute in
Cooperation with Tufts–
New England Medical Center*

THE MACMILLAN COMPANY, NEW YORK
COLLIER-MACMILLAN LTD., LONDON

To those who labor

to make drugs more effective

and less necessary

Contents

Preface

BOSTON was already a major city boasting a booming maritime economy in the early 1800's when John Lowell, Jr., conceived of the Lowell Institute and envisioned a series of lectures as its initial offering.

Even in 1840, however, the year the Lowell Lectures opened, Bostonians were still bound by the strictures of Puritanism, which forebade all worldly amusements including the legitimate theater. The only public relief from this rigid moralistic code came in the spirited oratory of the meeting house, which in fact provided as much entertainment as it did civic argument. Cast against today's standards it's easily understood why Puritanism now carries among its definitions "the haunting fear that someone, some-where, is enjoying himself."

Yet the founder of the institute was remarkably foresighted in setting the purpose of the lectures. In his will he stated: "As the prosperity of my native land, New England, which is sterile and unproductive, must depend hereafter as it has heretofore depended, first on the moral qualities and secondly on the intelligence and information of its inhabitants, I am desirous of trying to contribute toward this second object; and I wish courses of lectures to be established on physics and chemistry with their application to the arts, also on botany, zoology and mineralogy, connected with their particular utility to man."

And then he amended his directive to permit any future trustee freedom to exercise his own judgment to "from time to time establish lectures on any subject that in his opinion the wants and tastes of the age demand."

During the intervening years four distinguished members of the Lowell family have served as "corporation sole," the single trustee of the institute. The first trustee was John Amory Lowell, who had instituted banking policies in Boston that were so sound they weathered financial panics in 1837 and 1857. For the first lecture he chose Benjamin Silliman, a moving spirit in the founding of the medical school and later the father of science instruction at Yale, and the most eminent scientist of the day in the United States. What may have been Lowell's boldest stroke came, however, with his importing of the famed Swiss naturalist Louis Agassiz, who stayed on to become professor of zoology and geology at Harvard's new science school. "And in this arrangement American natural history at last found its leader," acknowledges Edward Weeks in his book *The Lowells and Their Institute*. The first litterateur selected to lecture was Dr. Oliver Wendell Holmes, though at this time his efforts were still primarily devoted to medicine. The invitation to deliver a course of lectures on English poets, Dr. Holmes later noted, resulted in "almost remaking my intellectual life." About this time trustee Lowell also was privately deeply involved in supporting the creation of a school of practical science, the Massachusetts Institute of Technology. Near the close of his stewardship and with the help of his son Augustus, who would become the second trustee, the lectures took on broader tone. For example a young doctor, William James, then teaching at Harvard, spoke on "The Brain and the Mind." And Oliver Wendell Holmes, Jr., gave twelve lectures on common law that summed up a decade of his work. Later he would be appointed to the Supreme Bench by President Theodore Roosevelt.

Augustus Lowell, one of the early industrial giants in the manufacture of textiles, took command of the institute in 1871 during the troubled aftermath of the Civil War. When the intensity of postwar feeling began to subside, the lectures provided a stage for military leaders to recount the critical army and navy battles and strategies in a reflective context, material later published for its historical value. By reinvesting a portion of the income, a practice continued by later trustees, Augustus increased the fund to a point where he could begin to carry out the secondary purpose of the will: to provide other courses on subjects in which college level instruction was needed. In one of his educational ventures he worked in conjunction with William Barton Rogers, then president of the fledgling Massachusetts Institute of Technology, to inaugurate evening courses, thus planting the seed of adult education in the United States. Near the close of the nineteenth century the lectures began to reflect America's growing curiosity about the Near and Far East. Other lectures introduced Russian history and literature, explored a new discovery, the X-ray, and a notable six-part series was given on "The Ethics of Marriage" by Professor Felix Adler.

A. Lawrence Lowell was himself a Lowell lecturer prior to his becoming the third trustee of the institute in 1902 at the age of forty-five. Seven years later he succeeded to the presidency of Harvard University. In both capacities he enlarged the programs within his jurisdiction. Rather than natural sciences, his interests ran to history and the arts though he never asked his younger sister, poetess Amy Lowell, to lecture. No woman ever had. A new flavor was added, however, in his choice of men from the "new" sciences. Among the Lowell lecturers in the first decade of the 1900's were Dr. James Putnam, who spoke on "Prevalent Nervous Derangements"; Professor Theodore Richards on "Early History and Recent Developments of Atomic Theory"; and Percival Lowell on "Mars as the Abode of Life." Via the institute, trustee Lowell merged the Lowell School of Practical Design with the Museum of Fine Arts. He consolidated the free courses at Massachusetts Institute of Technology into a two-year formal course. And he focused the main support of the institute on popular and adult education, arranging for university extension courses at Harvard, Boston University, Boston College, Tufts, Wellesley, and the Boston Museum of Fine Arts. At the close of his trusteeship the lectures grew even more brilliant, with the appearance of world figures such as historian Arnold Toynbee, philosopher Alfred North Whitehead, astronomer Harlow Shapley, and experimental zoologist Julian Huxley, who assessed "Man's Place in the Universe." Advance rumblings of World War II were heard in a series of lectures given on the collapse of the Weimar Republic, at about the same time the trusteeship of the institute again changed hands.

In 1938, when the present trustee of the Lowell Institute, Ralph Lowell, assumed the post, the public's lecture-going habit was going out of style. Attendance had fallen sharply, although it would peak now and again with the appearances of men like Bernard deVoto or Arthur Schlesinger, Jr. Meanwhile, the radio had been born and somewhat fatefully it was this new medium that would ensure the future of the Lowell Lectures. In the late 1940's Harvard president James B. Conant, reluctant to lead the university directly into the educational radio business, suggested the radio as a way out of both their problems to Harvard overseer Ralph Lowell. Out of their deliberations on October 6, 1951, came the Educational Foundation with its station WGBH-FM. Two years later, when TV channels became available, the foundation was awarded Channel 2 for WGBH for educational television use. The lectures thus could be broadcast and televised, expanding the audience to an extent impossible for the founder to have imagined. For lecturers Ralph Lowell sought modernists and contemporary subjects; ex-ambassador George F. Kennan to discuss "Russia and the West"; Dana L. Farnsworth on "Mental Health in Colleges and Universities"; McGeorge Bundy on "The Conservative in Modern American Politics." And the first woman Lowell lecturer was engaged, Cecilia Payne Goposchkin to discuss "Stellar Evolution." The lectures now were styled toward annual presentations in four fields: the arts, natural sciences, history or biography, and a symposium on contemporary medicine. Since their start in 1947 the medical lectures have drawn national authorities to the podium.

The following series of Lowell Lectures on "The Medicated Society" is the first under the sponsorship of the Tufts-New England Medical Center. The lectures were given weekly for twelve weeks beginning on January 16, 1967.

I am deeply indebted to the physicians of our own staff and to professional colleagues from major medical centers across the country who so willingly and ably participated in this Lowell Lecture series. In the success of the series, many others also played prominent and productive roles. Other members of Tufts-New England Medical Center staff who were of indispensable help were Donald K. Korth, Jr., Coordinator for Planning; Daniel S. Gillmor, Assistant to the Deans of Tufts University Schools of Medicine and Dental Medicine; Patricia G. Mazza, Public Relations Director and Director of Communications for the Lowell Lecture series; her assistant Rhoda Fischer; and Alice B. Millen, secretarial assistant to the series. A sincere expression of gratitude also is extended to WGBH-TV staff members, especially John Caldwell, Executive Producer of the Educational Division; Susan Hight, Producer of the Lowell Series; James Kelly, Assistant Director; and Harold Pyke, Jr., Project Coordinator. A final and special note of thanks goes to Boston medical writer Loretta McLaughlin, who served as manuscript editor.

Introduction

SAMUEL PROGER, M.D.

THE AMERICAN PUBLIC is said to be "drug happy," using enormous quantities of prescription drugs along with self-prescribed medicines ranging from aspirin and antacids to tranquilizers, rubbing compounds, and suppositories.

Approximately one billion prescriptions are filled annually in this country. This is double the number that were filled just ten years ago and represents about five prescriptions for every man, woman, and child. Some five thousand new prescription products were introduced in the 1950's (3,100 have since been replaced or improved). Then there are the nonprescription drugs. More than half of the drug purchases come over the open counter.

There are today more valid uses for drugs than ever before. Great advances in drug therapy account for some of the acceptable increase in drug usage. Some of the merited increase in drug usage can also be attributed to an increase in the aging population, a population that requires a more frequent use of drugs for maintenance therapy. But people seem to have become more disease conscious, and they seek medical aid for more trifling ailments, or they take drugs for no ailment at all.

In the eighteenth century, Benjamin Franklin could remark with good reason that there was very little difference between the

[1]

good doctor and no doctor. The good doctor, knowing the limitations of the medicines of his day, knew that he could do very little for most illnesses. But Franklin went on to say that there was a great difference between the good doctor and the bad doctor. The bad doctor, unaware of those limitations, proceeded to use treatments that were often harmful and occasionally even lethal. Unfortunately, there are many illnesses even today to which Franklin's remarks still apply; and while the modern physician can no longer be described as a "practitioner of ritual murder," we must in all candor recognize that patients are still suffering and dying unnecessarily as a consequence of the misuse of drugs.

The chapters that follow cover a broad range of topics and views. The first provides a historical framework in which to visualize our modern problems. The discussion of contraceptives illustrates the immense role that drugs can play as a beneficial social force, while the chapter on hallucinogens and narcotics offers noteworthy examples of the possible harmful social effects of drugs. The discussion of antibiotics furnishes a splendid opportunity to demonstrate the ideal in drug usage. In this respect the saga of the discovery, the development, the manufacture, and the distribution of antibiotics is a story without parallel in the history of medicine.

The consideration of what drugs may do to the unborn child raises troublesome questions. From time immemorial pregnant women have been taking drugs and various other substances with no awareness whatsoever of their possible effects on the fetus. We now know that these effects are many and diverse. Are there other such large dark areas still unexplored?

One of the more fascinating as well as more important areas of drug therapy is that related to mental illness. The current status of drugs in mental illness gives encouragement for the present and hope for the future. The same may be said of cancer.

Most people who live beyond middle age die of heart attacks

or strokes. In this area the preventive use of drugs probably has much to offer as indicated in discussion of this topic.

In another chapter we learn that drugs can produce as well as cure or ameliorate disease. Drug-induced illnesses are increasing in number. It behooves us to be aware of the nature and extent of this problem.

To learn more about the effects of drugs on man, we need to acquire knowledge of these actions in a manner that is both humane and scientific. There is no basic conflict between the scientific and the ethical approach to human drug testing, as indicated in the comments having to do with this subject.

The conflict between government and industry with respect to the use of drugs may prove to be more apparent than real. It is important that both points of view be understood, for then they can and surely will be reconciled. The chapters dealing with these viewpoints suggest that there is a large common ground of accommodation and collaboration.

Fads are so much a feature of therapy that we must always be on guard, lest we find ourselves unwittingly accepting popular remedies that are in fact nothing more than fashionable. There was a time when bleeding seemed to cure all actual or supposed illness. Then there was a period when purging was regarded as good for whatever ailed one. In the early part of this century most of man's illnesses were thought to be due to "auto intoxication." "Toxic" substances were not to be allowed to accumulate in the colon, lest we suffer dire consequences. As a result there was not only a veritable profusion of colonic irrigations, but respected surgeons were even removing colons in the belief that this was the most effective method of eliminating the harmful results of intestinal sluggishness. When we recovered from such folly, we entered upon an era during which "foci of infection" were believed to be the source of all medical troubles. Teeth were extracted, tonsils removed, prostates massaged, along with all manner of other intrusions, and all the while we were fully convinced not only of the logic of these procedures, but of their

benefits as well. We also recovered from this therapeutic binge
and then moved into a period when every illness was due to an
allergy of some sort. And then came the vitamin era. If there was
no definite evidence of vitamin deficiency, the lack was "subclini-
cal," that is to say it could not be demonstrated. It was there
nevertheless. Vitamins as a cure-all had at least the virtue of
being relatively harmless in the doses usually given.

Such enthusiasms appear irrational only in retrospect. They
seem quite reasonable during the period they are in favor. One
must be constantly on guard, therefore, against the subtle and
tyrannical influences of medical fashions. On the assumption that
we seem always to be immersed in some such fashion one must
ask oneself: What are we now doing in the treatment of patients
that to physicians a century hence will seem as quaint and often
as harmful as widespread bleeding and purging seem to us today?
Specifically one must ask: Is the excessive and otherwise improper use of drugs today's irrational fashion?

Drugs in one form or another have always been an important
part of man's life; they seem more important than ever today.
They occupy a large place in modern society. What appears to be
an overuse of drugs, however, comes at a time when we are in a
position to judge more adequately their beneficial and harmful
consequences. We are developing techniques of examination and
systems of controlled studies that enable us to determine drug
effects more accurately. We are acquiring much new information
about the actions of drugs, as, for example, on the unborn child.
We are coming to know something about how drugs in combination work. And we are more aware of the possible delayed, sometimes long-delayed, damaging effects of drugs.

In other words, as drugs are taken more widely and more
indiscriminately, scientists are providing more useful information, and at the same time government agencies are introducing
more regulatory controls. We appear to be in the midst of two
movements, both in full swing: the one leading to the improper
use of drugs, the other to corrective measures. Hopefully there

will result a balance, which will take us from the potential hazards of an unsuitably medicated society to the real benefits of an appropriately medicated society. To achieve this goal there must be a greater public awareness of the problems involved.

It was with this in mind that the following series of Lowell Lectures was conceived. The hope is that greater knowledge on the part of those who take drugs—that is all of us—will contribute to a more appropriate and more healthful application of the considerable advances in drug treatment to which we have fallen heir in recent years.

1

Drugs Through the Ages

LOUIS LASAGNA, M.D.

THE HISTORY OF MAN reveals an ancient preoccupation with the search for substances that might curtain off pain, salvage those bitten by the bloody jaws of war or fevered by contagion, and ease the agonies of the insane or the discomforts arising from bodies ravaged by age and disease. The story of this search is both fascinating and complex. In it are elements of genius and fraud, ignorance and nobility, logic and accident, self-sacrifice and self-aggrandizement. This story cries for a better historian and more extended treatment than are available to you in this chapter. In partial substitution, I plan to underscore some important *leit-motifs*—some dominant recurring themes—which must be appreciated if we are to profit from the successes and the failures of our predecessors.

Perhaps the most primitive theme is that of the anonymous folk remedy—the concoction derived from trial-and-error, monumental good luck, or some philosophical or magical concept. For example, a column from the Ebers papyrus reflects the medical procedures of at least a segment of Egyptian society some fifteen centuries or so before Christ. It contains the prescription for liver to treat night blindness, and it has directions for compounding over eight hundred prescriptions. Certain remedies seem eminently sensible even today—a number of obviously effective cathartics, for example—while others seem more naïve and of dubious efficacy. Yet even such a principle as the use of organs from numerous wild animals to treat disease of the corresponding human organ—swine eye for blindness is one such—has its modern counterpart in the use of animal thyroid or insulin from hog or beef pancreas to treat under-function of those endocrine glands in the human.

The origin of opium is lost in the thick gray fog of prehistory, but its power to bestow sleep, emotional tranquillity, and relief from pain has been treasured for many centuries. Opium is still harvested from the oriental poppy in a manner described by the Greek Dioscorides, a physician employed by Nero.

It is suspected that Homer was alluding to opium when he told about the drink that Helen gave in Sparta to Telemachus, Peisistratus, and Menelaus, to alleviate the gloomy atmosphere, when all were complaining that Odysseus had not yet come back. In the Odyssey we read:

Then Helen, daughter of Zeus, took other counsel. Straightaway she cast into the wine of which they were drinking a drug to quit all pain and strife, and bring forgetfulness of every ill. Whoso should drink this down, when it is mingled in the bowl, would not in the course of that day let a tear fall down over his cheeks, no, not though his mother and father should lie there dead, or though before his face men should slay with the sword his brother or dear son, and his own eyes behold it.

The search for drugs was unfortunately not then—or now—restricted to drugs helpful to mankind. Chemical warfare for example, which we tend to consider a modern conceit, was waged in the fifth century B.C. by the Spartans, who used burning sulphur and pitch to form sulphur dioxide in the siege of two Athenian cities. And there is, of course, the famous death of Socrates after quaffing a cup containing an extract of hemlock. In Plato's "Phaedo" there is the following passage:

With these words he put the cup to his lips and drank the poison quite calmly and cheerfully. Till then most of us had been able to control our grief fairly well; but when we saw him drinking, and then the poison finished, we could do so no longer: My tears came fast in spite of myself: It was not for him, but at my own misfortune in losing such a friend. . . . he walked about, until he said that his legs were getting heavy, and then he lay down on his back, as he was told. And the man who gave the poison began to examine his feet and legs, from time to time: Then he pressed his foot hard, and asked if there was any feeling in it; and Socrates said, No: And then his legs, and so higher and higher, and showed us that he was cold and stiff. And Socrates felt himself, and said that when it came to his heart, he should be gone. . . .

This report gives a reliable picture of the effects of the alkaloid coniine, the active constituent of the hemlock, to wit, paralysis of motor and sensory nerve endings and the central nervous system, with death following from poisoning of the respiratory center.

Many of the ancient folk-remedies were thought to be possessed of such broad curative powers that one cannot read of their alleged virtues with a straight face. Note the description of "garlick" in the seventeenth century herbal of Dr. Nicholas Culpeper:

It provokes urine, and women's courses, helps the biting of mad dogs and other venomous creatures [an unhappily ambiguous statement!], kills worms in children, cuts and voids tough phlegm, purges the head, helps the lethargy, is a good preservative against, and a remedy for any plague, sore, or foul ulcers; takes away spots and blemishes in the skin, eases pains in the ears, ripens and breaks . . . swellings. . . . It is also good in hydropick diseases, the jaundice, falling sickness, cramps, convulsions, the piles or haemorrhoids, or other cold diseases. . . . In coleric men it will add fuel to the fire; in men oppressed by melancholy, it will attenuate the humor, and send . . . strange visions to the head; therefore let it be taken inwardly with great moderation; outwardly you may make more bold with it.

The second *leitmotif* is that of the talented individual who single-handedly made a lasting contribution to the pharmacopeia, either by performing the crucial animal experiments or isolating the specific chemical from its plant, animal, or mineral source, or by convincing the world of truths long apparent to a few, but lying dormant outside the world's stream of consciousness.

One such person was James Lind, a Scottish ship's surgeon who performed a remarkably sophisticated experiment in 1747 aboard the British ship Salisbury. He took some sailors with scurvy, who were bedded together in one place and had one diet common to all. He treated two each with some suggested remedies for the disease: cider, elixir of vitriol, vinegar, sea water; an electuary of garlic, mustard, balsam of Peru and myrrh; and oranges and lemons. The effects with the last treatment were so dramatic that the benefits of citrus fruits were clearly demonstrated. (It nevertheless was a half century before an admiralty order finally prescribed lime juice for all hands, so that British sailors could become "limeys," and scurvy could eventually disappear from the Royal Navy.)

William Withering, an eighteenth century English physician, was another such pioneer. A competent botanist, who had written on "All the Vegetables Naturally Growing in Great Britain," he pursued with skill and imagination a complex old wives' remedy from Shropshire, which was allegedly good for patients with dropsy. His botanical interests led him to suspect that the multiple ingredients were not all necessary, and some shrewd detective work quickly revealed that the essential drug was to be found in the foxglove plant. Thus was begun one of the major advances in the treatment of heart failure, which eventually culminated in the isolation of purified digitalis glycosides a century later.

The scientist willing to venture forth into the pitiless spotlight of public controversy has played his role in the history of drugs no less than in other arenas of medical science. James Young Simpson, Professor of Obstetrics at Edinburgh in the nineteenth century and a pioneer in the investigation of chloroform, was faced with strong opposition to anesthesia, especially from a theologically oriented group of physicians and laymen, who objected to anesthesia as contrary to the wishes of God. In 1847

Simpson wrote a paper in which he utilized eloquence, a sound biblical background and knowledge of Hebrew, and tight reasoning to argue in favor of anesthetic agents in mid-wifery. After a skillful discussion of the original Hebrew word for "sorrow" in the phrase "in sorrow thou shalt bring forth children," Simpson delivered the coup de grace by quoting from the description in Genesis of "the first surgical operation ever performed on man": "And the Lord God caused a deep sleep to fall upon Adam; and he slept; and he took one of his ribs, and closed up the flesh instead thereof." Simpson further strengthened his case by quoting Calvin: "It ought to be noted that Adam was sunk into a profound sleep, in order that he might feel no pain."

Unfortunately, the contributions of individuals to drug development have not always been of the admirable variety. Pharmacology has its tawdry pages as well as its shining ones. In the seventeenth century, word is said to have gone from Lima to Spain that on the eastern slopes of the Andes a tree had been found, the bark of which cured malaria. The useful part of the tree became known as Jesuit's powder, because the members of this order were active in trying to popularize usage of the material. An English quack named Robert Talbor started to treat cases of malaria very successfully with a "secret" remedy in the 1660's, and in 1672 published a little book on his cure. He gave himself the title of "healer of fevers" and referred to a specific which he had for curing all sorts of agues, but never published any details of this remedy. Even Charles II was cured by Talbor, who was knighted and appointed physician to the King. He then went to the French Court, where he soon changed his name to Talbot, and cured of fever the Dauphin and other members of the Royal Family, as well as the Queen of Spain and numerous courtiers. The secret was bought by Louis XIV under the condition that it should not be divulged before the death of Talbor. Eventually the secret remedy was revealed to be the cinchona bark, the very Jesuit's powder of the New World. By order of King Louis, a booklet on the remedy was published in 1682 by a distinguished French surgeon and physician of the Court.

The controversy over ether anesthesia was even more sordid. After the successful and dramatic demonstration in the operating amphitheatre of the Massachusetts General Hospital, Morton, a dentist, and Jackson, a physician and chemist, fought for the right to fame and wealth as the original discoverers of ether. Morton and Jackson first tried, unsuccessfully, to patent ether. Later Jackson wrote to the French Academy of Sciences and announced himself alone to be the discoverer. Morton thereupon claimed this honor as rightly his own. A bitter series of verbal and written exchanges followed, and none of the leading characters emerged with honor untarnished. Indeed most of them were destined to end their lives under tragic circumstances.

The capacity of drugs to act as two-edged swords is well demonstrated by the story of cocaine, whose origins hark back to the chewing of coca leaves by South American Indians. In 1884 came an electrifying announcement from Vienna to the effect that painless surgery was possible by the use of cocaine as a local anesthetic. Dr. Carl Koller, an associate of Dr. Sigmund Freud, noticed that if one put a drop or two of a dilute solution of cocaine on the tip of one's tongue, tastelessness and insensibility followed almost immediately, later to disappear. Placing a few drops of a weak solution of cocaine in the eye of a guinea pig, Koller quickly found that even rough probing of the eye brought no response. Having heard many screaming patients at the Vienna Hospital, he naturally considered operations on the eye to be a perfect choice for investigation, as they represented excruciating ordeals not suitable for general anesthesia. He tried cocaine on a patient scheduled for removal of a cataract, and the removal was accomplished painlessly.

The depressing part of the story arises from Sigmund Freud's well meaning but unfortunate suggestion that cocaine injections might be useful in many kinds of psychiatric illness. Freud lived to see his hope turn to horror as cocaine addiction captured just those individuals whom he had hoped to cure with its use. In his autobiography the famous psychiatrist penned a revealing passage, which contains an amazingly transparent resentment about his failure to be present at the time his colleague (whom he later used to refer to facetiously as "Coca Koller") was performing the famous experiments. Freud had taken off to see his fiancée in Hamburg, and in his faulty recollection of the event not only mistakenly took credit for suggesting the possibility of using cocaine as a local anesthetic, but ends with the revealing phrase: ". . . but I bore my fiancée no grudge for her interruption of my work."(!)

The third recurring theme might be called "the profit-motif." There is of course nothing new about the desire for economic gain, and such urges have motivated men in a search for marketable drugs. The most popular prescription of the Middle Ages was something called theriacum. A whole library has been written on this medicine, which contained a large number of drugs, with the exact composition varying from time to time and place to place. The basic ingredient seems to have been viper flesh, but at one time the magic mishmash contained fifty-seven substances, and its preparation was considered so difficult that fifteenth-century Venice insisted it be made in the presence of certain authoritative physicians and pharmacists. It made money for a good many people, as did a rival preparation oroietan, which also provided Venice with a bonanza in trade.

Regardless of one's philosophy about the profit motive, it is hard to deny that it has yielded medical profits for mankind. Take, for example, the contribution of industry to the development of penicillin and other antibiotics. After the pioneer work by such nonindustrial scientists as Fleming and Waksman, the problem of producing pure antibiotics in bulk and distributing them all over the world was assumed by business firms unquestionably concerned with showing a profit at the end of the year. Such accomplishments might conceivably have been equaled by universities or a socialized drug industry, but the fact is that they were not.

Contrast the current situation in Indonesia, where the once orderly and businesslike devotion of Dutch colonialists to the

growing of Cinchona plants had provided the world with a steady
supply of quinine and quinidine. Java is no longer capable of
providing these drugs, and the result has been patients deprived
of important antimalarial therapy and a standard plant medication for the management of disorders of heart rhythm. Patients as
far apart as soldiers in Vietnam and cardiacs on the East Coast
of the United States have had occasion to feel the bite of the
worldwide shortage of these Cinchona products.

For several years it has been perpetual open season for sniping
at drug houses. In part, the pharmaceutical industry has asked
for such criticism by shoddy performance in the past. In part
also, the industry probably has suffered resentment because of
the power and success of modern drug houses. Not only have
drug firms made tremendous profits in the last twenty years, but
by their advertising and "educational" techniques they have
guided the practice of medicine in a way that is galling to those
who would like to see such guidance come from groups less likely
to have a bias arising out of the need to earn money for stock-
holders.

A fourth motif running throughout our story is that of social
control of drugs. In contrast to the antiquity of public interest in
drugs, public control of drugs is a relative newcomer to the scene.
The British Food and Drug Act, for example, was passed in 1872,
while in our own country effective legislative concern with this
problem did not begin until the twentieth century. Despite some
magnificent muckraking by such journalists as Samuel Hopkins
Adams, the evils of the patent medicine business were first
brought under legal surveillance because of public horror over a
novel entitled *The Jungle* by the then obscure socialist Upton
Sinclair. In its pages he described in horrible detail the filthy
conditions under which American meat was processed. Theodore Roosevelt and Congress were incensed, meat sales fell by
half, and the omnibus Pure Food and Drugs Act was passed.

Some three decades later the Food, Drug, and Cosmetic Act
became law, again because of public outrage over a specific dra-

matic incident—the Elixir of Sulfonilamide disaster. One hundred and seven people, many of them children, were fatally poisoned by the diethylene glycol in which a small southern firm had dissolved the new miracle drug. The solvent had been tested for appearance, flavor, and fragrance, but not for safety.

A quarter of a century later the cycle was repeated, as the thalidomide tragedy exploded on the pages of the world's news media. This drug, which appeared almost inert in animals, had proved capable of deforming babies carried by women who had taken the mild sedative early in pregnancy. The fact that the incident had little or nothing to do with most of the substance of the Kefauver-Harris Amendments was beside the point; public pressures had once again transformed an apathetic Congress into indignant, crusading public defenders. The Senate and the House, some of whose members can almost always find reasons to object to legislation, voted unanimously to pass the bill.

Today the public is once again alarmed about drugs—narcotics, marihuana, barbiturates, amphetamines, LSD. None of these agents are new, but the flood of journalistic accounts, the increasing use of drugs by students, beatniks, and psychiatric fringe elements, and the evangelical exhortations of psychedelic messiahs, who find God in their novels and Eternal Truth in hallucinations and perceptual distortions, have aroused the sleepy legislative beasts and brought about a spate of restrictive and punitive legislation, some of it reasonable, some of it excessive and ill-considered.

A fifth *leitmotif* in the history of drugs is the clinical point-counter-point between uncontrolled, chance observations and rigorous experimentation. Progress in science has in general been considerably more rapid when scientists have performed true experiments, *i.e.,* have purposely manipulated variables in a systematic manner, rather than rely on random observations of naturally occurring phenomena. While one can read in the Book of Daniel about control groups utilized to study the effects of diet on the well-being of some subjects of King Nebuchadnezzar, the notion of controls—in the sense of check or test observations to provide a standard of comparison—did not really come into scientific parlance until relatively late in the nineteenth century, despite earlier attempts by David Hume and John Stuart Mill to lay down rules for experimental inquiry. In therapeutics, however, the widespread use of control groups has been a development of the past three decades.

This development has paralleled changes in the science of statistics. Originally, all statistics were really historic, concerned with a recording of the past. In time, however, due to the development of sampling techniques and the introduction of other statistical concepts, statistics became very much concerned with the present, with the comparison of measurements, and the projection of such comparisons, on the basis of probability theory, to members of the population other than those actually studied.

There is no question but that most of our therapeutic advances over the centuries have not been the result of controlled experimentation. Many useful drugs have evolved in an unplanned, helter-skelter way. On the other hand many duds have also been "discovered" in this way. The literature is replete with hundreds of "cures" for hypertension, alcoholism, cancer, diabetes, etc., which have failed the test of time. In my medical school years, for example, chaulmoogra oil was considered the standard method of therapy for leprosy. Today, this material is generally held to be inert therapeutically, yet for decades lepers were injected with chaulmoogra oil in the mistaken belief that the progress of the disease was retarded in some way, even if cures were not achieved.

What are the lessons from this brief review of the past? The first is that we must not neglect folk remedies and natural materials, since the latter constitute about half of our prescribed drugs. There are said to be several hundred thousand plant species, of which only some twenty thousand have been screened to any degree for pharmacological activity. Perhaps the most exciting story in recent years in regard to folk remedies is that of the periwinkle plant, which was investigated because it was considered to be a folk remedy for diabetes. Investigation in animals seemed to indicate that the drug did not have any effect on blood sugar, but the animals were noted to die of what appeared to be overwhelming infection. Further inquiry showed that the animals were dying of infection because their white blood cell formation had been depressed by the periwinkle brew. Since this kind of effect is a hallmark of anti-cancer drugs, extracts of periwinkle were tried in patients with cancer, and today at least two purified materials from the periwinkle are proving highly successful in treating Hodgkin's disease as well as a malignant tumor of placental origin called choriocarcinoma, and some cases of acute leukemia.

The periwinkle story also reminds us that we must not turn up our noses at happy accidents. In 1869 Liebreich was convinced that chloral hydrate should be an effective hypnotic drug because it would be converted in the body to chloroform, a known central nervous system depressant. This theory is now known to be completely wrong. Chloral hydrate is *not* metabolized in this way, but the fact remains that chloral hydrate was and is one of our most trusted sleep-inducing agents. The happy accident of a mold settling on some culture medium and inhibiting the growth of bacterial colonies growing on the plate was not ignored by Alexander Fleming, who had the "prepared mind" required to take advantage of such a happy accident. Nonetheless, we must simultaneously pursue the evaluation of drugs systematically and in impeccable experimental fashion, whenever possible. Luck and reason need not be mutually exclusive.

Another lesson is that we cannot afford to do without the contributions of individual nonindustrial or academic researchers. Paradoxically, the very success of the pharmaceutical industry has deluded many scientists into believing that no one outside of a huge industrial complex can possibly contribute to the search for new drugs. Have these misguided dons so quickly forgotten the origins of penicillin, streptomycin, the use of antimetabolites in leukemia and gout, the antithyroid drugs, and cortisone? Where would these drugs have come from without Fleming, Waksman, Farber, Rundles, Astwood, and Kendall? Would those monastic university scientists who sneer at "applied" research not feel their faculties graced by a Paul Ehrlich? This German genius, with his brilliant and probing mind, opened up the whole field of chemotherapy with his "magic bullet" concept and his contributions to the treatment of trypanosomiasis and syphilis. Indeed his theoretical considerations of cell-drug interactions remain the foundation of modern work on cell receptor theory. The rational search for new drugs—depending as it does on hard-headed logic, rigorous scientific method, and an intimate knowledge of both disease mechanisms and drug action—calls for the highest level of intellectual dedication and ability. It may be too difficult for most of us, but it is certainly not second-class science.

These remarks should not be interpreted as a denigration of the role of the drug industry. Its financial resources are enormous, its ranks filled with many talented scientists. Were its creative contribution nil—and it is not—the existence of drug houses would be justified by their function as accoucheurs of new drugs —technological obstetricians delivering the end product safely from its source to the outside world. Yet the goals of society and of industry will never be isomorphic. No business can be run as a philanthropic research foundation, and profits and the public weal may at times compete for the loyalties of the men in the drug industry. To me, therefore, it seems inevitable that society must exercise some form of control over the sale and use of drugs.

Whether such control is optimal in the United States at present is doubtful. Many feel that our system is bogged down in bureaucratic inefficiency, and some have suggested that we might take a page from the infinitely simple British system. Whatever the best solution may be, society cannot afford impasses or obstructionism in this area anymore than it can afford reckless, irresponsible, or premature regulatory actions. The recent publicity over patient consent in clinical trials has triggered shrill demands for restrictions which not only ignore certain fundamental aspects of the patient-doctor relationship but also promise to prevent completely some kinds of research. No one wishes to trample on the rights of human beings, but it would be cruel indeed to trade theoretic civil libertarian gains for actual public harm through failure to develop new drugs or keep useless drugs off the market.

We must also keep reminding ourselves of the need for humility. We are ignorant about so many things. Our brothers in centuries past could not be efficient in their use of quinine because the words "fever" and "ague" covered such a mass of conditions that malaria was lost in obscure semantics. All credit to Withering, but it is not possible to read his classic work on digitalis without realizing how handicapped he was by the mysteries of "dropsy." It took years of investigation on the nature of edema, heart disease, and cardiac irregularities to allow modern rationale to evolve—and even now we are not certain about the mode of action of digitalis, to say nothing of such other ancient remedies as aspirin and morphine. How deluded are we today? How many wrong medical things are we doing, thinking, writing, saying? Are not "hypertension," "cancer," "depression" likely to be as scorned by the doctor of 2100 as "dropsy" and "ague" are by us? (This is not to say that we need be paralyzed by our ignorance. After all, Jenner discovered vaccination before anyone knew viruses existed. Nor does knowing the cause of a disease guarantee that we will be able to figure out a cure, I might add.)

The last quarter century has witnessed a revolution in therapeutics. It has been marked by the introduction of many important drugs—chemicals that have eased the suffering and increased the comfort of millions of patients, and have saved the lives of both young and old. One has but to list some of these advances to appreciate the gains. The sulfonamides, penicillin, chloramphenicol, streptomycin, isoniazid, and other chemotherapeutic agents have altered the natural course of meningitis, pneumonia, tuberculosis, and typhoid fever and tamed these ancient killers. The patient undergoing surgery today has the benefit of new anesthetics and muscle relaxants during the operation and of new potent pain-killers afterward. The child with leukemia is no longer doomed to the horrible, rapidly deteriorating course that was the rule twenty-five years ago. The patient with malignant hypertension, once almost certain to die within a year or two after onset of his disease, now has powerful drugs to control the effects of high blood pressure. The patient with Addison's disease can now live a life that is essentially normal and less hazardous than that of the average diabetic.

But the very accomplishments are deceptive. They suggest to the public that we have solved most of the serious disease problems threatening us. In fact, we are almost powerless to treat most cancers, or coronary or cerebral atherosclerosis. Our drugs for rheumatoid arthritis are all limited in efficacy and disturbing in their side effects, and none is curative. Our mental hospitals and chronic disease homes are full of patients who have reason to be dissatisfied with the miracle drugs of today. We have little to offer either the obese or the alcoholic. The public has a right to demand continued progress in the pharmaceutical fight against disease.

But the discovery of new drugs is not enough. The best drug is useless if not prescribed and dangerous if misused. The medical profession and the public both must be kept up-to-date on new drugs and on new information about old drugs, including when not to use them. Here are two relevant quotations for physicians anxious to avoid the image portrayed in this eighteenth century caricature:

"It is an easy matter to know the effects of honey, wine, hellebore, cautery, and cutting. But to know how, for whom, and when we should apply these . . . is no less an undertaking than being a physician"—(Aristotle).

"For, in diseases of the mind, as well as in other ailments, it is an art of no little importance to administer medicines properly:

but, it is an art of much greater and more difficult acquisition to know when to suspend or altogether to omit them"—(Philippe Pinel).

And here are two other quotations, which are especially interesting in view of the title of this series of Lowell Lectures and a recent survey by the Stanford Research Institute, which sampled medicine chests in San Francisco and found that an average of 29.5 medications was contained in each:

"To take no medicine is as good as a middling doctor"—(Chinese proverb).

"One of the first duties of the physician is to educate the masses not to take medicine"—(Sir William Osler).

There is much that we need to know. How do our drugs work? How do they interact with other drugs to produce serious toxicity or to potentiate each other's beneficial effects? How much do people differ in their handling of drugs, and how far do such interpatient differences in metabolism go to explain the tremendous variability in dosage required to produce therapeutic effects or toxicity? How do children differ from adults in their response to drugs? What genetic factors are important in determining drug effects? Why do some drugs lose their effect on continued use? How can we better tailor drugs to specific patients, picking drugs in advance rather than relying on trial and error techniques? What are the most effective ways of administering drugs, in terms of route of administration, timing of doses, etc.? How can we better predict human toxicity—including that on the fetus—from animal studies? How can we detect serious toxicity early in the career of a drug? How can one prove cause-and-effect relationship in drug reactions reliably and with a minimum of risk to the public?

In order best to understand the mysteries of therapeutics, we must also study what might be called the sociology of drug usage. Why do some patients fail to fill prescriptions? Why do so many fail to follow the doctor's directions? How can we decrease medication errors by pharmacists and nurses? What determines a physician's choice between alternative drugs? Where do doctors acquire their information (and misinformation) about therapeutic agents? What form should advertisements take to provide the right kind of information to the prescribing physician? How can doctors be taught to evaluate the drug literature? How much disagreement is there between doctor and patient in regard to the goals and achievements of drug therapy? What should the doctor and patient know about the economics of drug production and distribution?

This, then, has been one clinical pharmacologist's view of "Drugs Through The Ages." You may remember the story told by Cicero of Damocles, who was horrified, while sitting in the chair of the tyrant Dionysius of Syracuse, to see hanging over him a sword suspended by a single hair. The tale has become a symbol of the catastrophe threatening even those who seem most secure and in positions of great power.

Modern drugs possess great power for good, but this power is accompanied by the risk of great dangers. There are hazards from drug effects per se and less tangible hazards ranging from inequitable or punitive social strictures on industry or the medical profession to the harm that can come from failure to discover new agents so badly needed to treat the diseases that afflict us. It is impossible for me to imagine a time when men will be able to reap the benefits of powerful chemicals without paying some price, suffering some loss. The job facing us is maximizing the benefits while minimizing the risks. This effort will require the talents, interest, and good will of laboratory scientists, physicians, businessmen, politicians, regulatory agencies, and the consumers. We might begin our journey by agreeing that the goal we wish to reach is not a "medicated society" but a healthy society.

NOTE ON CONTRIBUTOR

Louis Lasagna (M.D. 1947, College of Physicians and
Surgeons, Columbia University), is head of the Division of
Clinical Pharmacology and associate professor of medicine
and associate professor of pharmacology and experimental
therapeutics, Johns Hopkins University School of Medicine, Baltimore, Maryland. He serves on the editorial
boards of the *Journal of Chronic Diseases, Journal of
Psychiatric Research, Methods of Medical Information,*
and *Psychopharmacologia.* He is also consultant to the
National Institute of General Medical Sciences and the
National Heart Institute.

2

The Abuse of Hallucinogens and Opiates

DONALD B. LOURIA, M.D. (F.A.C.P.)

THROUGHOUT HISTORY MAN has sought surcease from the rigors of an all too frequently unfriendly environment. At times escape has been achieved by participation in self-hypnotizing, religious, or pseudoreligious rituals, and at times by the use of potent hallucinogens. Thus, in Mexico, archaeological evidence suggests that use and worship of hallucinogenic mushrooms can be traced as far back as 1500 B.C. Similarly, chewing of the hallucinogenic cactus, peyote, has been practiced many hundreds of years in North America. In Australia, aborigines perform prodigious feats of strength under the influence of pituri, which contains several potent alkaloids including scopolamine. Several Siberian tribes use mushrooms containing the hallucinogens muscarine and bufotine. Natives of the Amazon, to prepare themselves for brutal whipping ceremonies, drink caapi, the active hallucinogenic component of which is banisterene. In certain areas of Africa, ibogaine, a harmine-like alkaloid, is the hallucinogen used, and in India a variety of cannabis provides hallucinatory escape. Thus it is the world over—man utilizes drugs to escape the unpleasantness of reality.

[23]

In the United States our traditional escape from the real or imagined travails of life has been through ingestion of alcohol. Among the 20 per cent of Americans living in poverty there is no apparent community acceptance of either hallucinogenic or narcotic drugs as an alternative to alcohol. There are two major exceptions to this: First, among the Plains Indians, many of whom endure grinding poverty, peyote is used extensively and legally in intermittent religious ceremonies under the aegis of the Native American Church; and second at least 80 per cent of heroin abusers reside in areas of urban blight. In certain subsections of New York City, the use of heroin has almost gained community acceptance as an escape mechanism.

Although the 20 per cent who do not share American affluence do not generally abuse potent hallucinogens, an increasing number of the 80 per cent who share in society's material well being do.

The major potent hallucinogens used in the United States today and their sources are listed in Table 1.

TABLE 1

Potent hallucinogens illicitly used in United States	Source
Lysergic acid diethylamide-LSD-25	Mushroom
Psilocybin	Mushroom
Mescaline	Cactus
Dimethyltryptamine (DMT)	Readily synthesized
Bufotenine (rarely used)	Mushroom
Hashish (pure cannabis resin)	Cannabis sativa (plant)

Of these, the best known and most frequently abused is lysergic acid diethylamide (LSD-25). Synthesized in 1938, its hallucinogenic properties were inadvertently discovered five years later. In the intervening twenty-four years, a farrago of well over fifteen hundred articles has appeared in the medical and para-medical literature analyzing the sociological, physiological, pharmacological, psychological, and biochemical effects of LSD in experimental animals and man.

It now appears that LSD, given under careful medical surveillance, may be potentially beneficial in the following six circumstances.

Chronic alcoholism. In various series, 20 to 60 per cent of those suffering from severe alcoholism improved markedly after one to three administrations of LSD, improvement being defined as abstinence or striking reduction in alcohol consumption. These studies, although a cause for optimism, are not entirely convincing. Frequently the follow-up period has been inadequate and adscititious rehabilitative measures have precluded a judgment concerning the specific role of LSD.

Sexual abnormalities. A small number of patients suffering from sexual abnormalities, especially homosexuality and frigidity, have been treated with LSD with encouraging results in a few cases. Here, too, the data are currently far too meager.

Schizophrenic children. Ordinarily schizophrenia, or even a severely schizoid personality, constitutes an absolute contraindication to LSD treatment. In children, however, LSD may effect improvement after many other therapeutic measures fail.

Psychoneurosis. In psychotherapy, LSD may be beneficial in some patients with neuroses, especially those characterized by compulsions and obsessions. Enough patients have been so treated to establish as valid the use of the drug in carefully selected cases.

Psychopaths. In one series, 14 of 21 psychopaths benefited strikingly from LSD, but the data are clearly insufficient.

Terminal disease. LSD is a potent analgesic. When given to patients suffering from painful and inexorably progressive malignant disease, LSD alleviated the pain and in some provided equanimity in the face of imminent death.

These potential medical uses establish LSD as a drug that might in the future be of immense benefit to the medical profession. With LSD the problem arises not from its potential medical uses but from its indiscriminate use by those outside the medical profession. The questions that arise then concern the nature of the dangers, the incidence of abuse, and possible remedial measures.

It is first mandatory to outline the putative wonders and ecstasies of LSD. Some years ago Aldous Huxley capsulized the potential glories of potent hallucinogens.

Pharmacology has now entered upon a period of rapid growth, and it seems quite certain that in the next few years scores of new methods for changing the quality of consciousness will be discovered. The pharmacologist will give us something that most human beings have never had before. They will give us loving kindness, peace and joy. If we want beauty, they will transfigure the outside world for us and open the door to visions of unimaginable riches and significance. If our desire is for life everlasting, they will give us the next best thing; aeons of blissful experience miraculously telescoped into a single hour. They will bestow these gifts without exacting the terrible price that, in the past, men had to pay for resorting too frequently to such consciousness-changing drugs as heroin or cocaine, or even that good old standby, alcohol. Already we have at our disposal hallucinogens and tranquilizers whose physiological price is amazingly low and there seems to be every reason to believe that the consciousness changers, the tension-relievers of the future, will do their work even more efficiently and at even lower cost to the individual. Human beings will be able to achieve effortlessly what in the past could only be achieved with difficulty by means of self-control and spiritual exercises.

Once LSD is taken, an orgy of brilliant visual images occurs: These may be beautiful, bizarre, terrifying, or have a religious connotation. Auditory hallucinations may also occur. The recent claims that LSD is a powerful physical aphrodisiac are controverted by the experience of virtually every responsible investigator in the field. Whatever LSD may or may not be, it does not generally act as an aphrodisiac. The power of the experience almost ineluctably leads to claims of striking personal benefit and new productivity. The claims of productivity are usually related to artistic achievement: Since this is a subjective area, it is virtually impossible to make any valid judgment. However, three pieces of data suggest the claims often are egregiously exaggerated. First, psychiatrists experienced in the use of LSD note that they frequently cannot substantiate their patients' claims concerning LSD benefits. Second, a study on ten patients with sexual perversions showed improvement in two; regarding the others, the authors wrote, "the impression gained is that whilst they usually claim to be improved, the improvement is not confirmed by subsequent behavior." This is an important observation because the subjective feelings could readily be checked against the pre- and post-treatment sexual behavior patterns. Third, the experience at Bellevue Hospital in New York City indicates that in a group of patients hospitalized with LSD-induced psychoses, the claims of improvement for the most part could not be substantiated by careful psychological or psychiatric examination.

In regard to the foregoing, then, in summary, LSD produces beneficial results in carefully selected patients treated under strict medical supervision. Taken in less controlled circumstances, LSD engenders ecstatic claims, but there is little evidence to suggest lasting benefit.

If one accepts the validity of the notion that prolonged benefits are infrequent when LSD is taken under nonmedical aegis, then the major question facing society and the potential user is the nature and extent of serious undesirable reactions.

The experience at Bellevue Hospital first detailed by Frosch, Robbins, and Stern, which has been subsequently confirmed elsewhere, documents vividly the potential dangers of illicitly taken LSD. During the past eighteen months more than 130 patients have been hospitalized with LSD-induced acute psychoses or with chronic schizophrenia (or schizoid personality) exacerbated by LSD ingestion. The characteristics of these are summarized in Table 2.

TABLE 2

Some characteristics of 114 LSD users

Average age	23 (range 15-43)
Male	68.4%
White	88.4%
LSD 1-3 times only	72.8%
Overwhelming panic	13.1%
Violence	12.3%
Homicidal or suicidal	8.6%
Underlying overt mental disease	34.2%
Requiring extended hospitalization	15.8%

Of the 114, 13.1 per cent suffered profound terror, 12.3 per cent exhibited uncontrolled violence, and 8.6 per cent attempted either homicide or suicide. Extended hospitalization was needed for 15.8 per cent, and of these almost half had no prior history of mental illness. The overwhelming majority had taken LSD on only one to three occasions. Interestingly, 88.4 per cent were white: Negro and Puerto Rican ethnic groups, which constitute approximately 25 per cent of the New York City population, provided only 11.6 per cent of the cases of LSD intoxication. Of the 114, 34 per cent had clear evidence of severe, pre-existing personality disturbances.

Of the 114 cases, a clear statement was made concerning occupation in 68. These are listed in Table 3. A substantial number of the patients were clearly from the middle or upper class economic groups and were of average to above average intelligence.

TABLE 3

Occupational history 68 cases	
Student	15
High school	6
College or graduate	9
Unemployed	12
Writer, artist, musician, photographer	11
Cook, waiter, caterer	7
Welder, carpenter, printer	5
Model, dancer	5
Physician, engineer, pharmacist	4
Sociologist, teacher	4
Typist, beautician	2
Housewife	2
Rancher	1

In some of the cases, dramatic untoward reactions to the drug occurred.

—A young man, in a panic, jumped from a fourth floor window fracturing many bones.

—A college student under the influence of LSD had a two-inch chunk of tissue taken out of his cheek by a friend, also under the influence of LSD. The former has since required extensive plastic surgery.

—A young man tried to kill the two-year-old child of his girl friend.

—A man jumped in front of a train because LSD-induced voices told him to do so. Fortunately, he escaped serious injury.

—A young woman in an LSD panic was found naked, incoherent, and violent, wandering around the streets at night.

There can then be no doubt that LSD can induce acute psychosis in an apparently healthy person, and it can decompensate a compensated or borderline schizophrenic, resulting in prolonged institutionalization. Furthermore, LSD-induced hallucinations may return days or even weeks after LSD ingestion if the individual is placed in a stressful situation. This may happen even if no LSD is taken in the interim. Although no homicidal or suicidal acts were carried out successfully among our patients, an increasing number of suicides and at least one homicide have occurred under the drug's influence.

Indeed the data documenting the extraordinary dangers of LSD appear virtually incontrovertible. The only remaining question is whether a previously "normal" person can have a psychotic reaction which results in either long-term hospitalization or permanent deleterious mental effects. This question at present remains unanswered. The profound effects of LSD on the nervous system and the phenomenon of late recurrence of the experience without further ingestion suggest that the drug might well permanently alter, for better or for worse, the personality structure of the individual. Further, the potency of the drug suggests that if permanent changes occur, only a single experience with LSD may be needed. If such potentially long-standing adverse effects do occur, the group most likely to be so affected are those given LSD without their own knowledge. This is a reprehensible act for the recipient almost uniformly reacts to the unexpected distortions of reality and hallucinations with fear, agitation, confusion, and at times overwhelming and terrifying panic.

There are additional problems with LSD.

First, there is increasing evidence that repeated or chronic use establishes a form of psychopathology not found if the drug is taken one to three times or only infrequently. The chronic user becomes immersed in the ramifications of hallucinogenic drug use, withdraws from the usual activities of society and in conventional terms becomes nonproductive. Thus far this drug-induced withdrawal from and indifference to society involves only a small number of persons. If, however, the abuse of LSD becomes more widespread, if more of the illicit users become involved in frequent use of LSD, then the dangers are immense of creating a substantial subsegment of society which does not participate in or contribute to society, devoting its total efforts instead to increasing the size of the drug subculture.

Second, the Bellevue Hospital experience suggests that an increasing percentage of the LSD abusers have marked underlying personality disturbances. The deluge of uncritical, often specious publicity and the miraculous effects attributed to LSD use by its proponents are influencing susceptible, unstable individuals to seek their own psychological salvation by self-administration of LSD under uncontrolled or inadequately supervised conditions. There is, as noted above, no evidence that taking LSD under such circumstances is beneficial, and in some cases this results in profound mental deterioration necessitating prolonged psychiatric hospitalization. In these individuals, prolonged or even permanent harm can result.

Third, LSD apparently can cause chromosomal aberrations, raising the specter of severe genetic damage. Thus far, *in vitro* and three of five *in vivo* studies of circulating human white blood cells show a striking increase in chromosomal breaks. Furthermore, chromosomal rearrangements, a genetically highly important abnormality, have been described. The chromosomal abnormalities are not strictly dose-related but in general occur more frequently if there is repeated exposure to more than 200 micrograms. The changes appear to persist after LSD administration is discontinued, and children born of LSD-using mothers may show chromosomal defects; these, too, appear to persist. Whether these chromosomal abnormalities will be associated with physical or mental defects in the users or their progeny is not yet known and will require epidemiologic research over a two-generation period to make a definitive judgment. But the potential genetic dangers of LSD are so great that this alone should cause many young persons to reject the blandishments of the drug proselytizers.

The incidence of LSD abuse and adverse reactions to it are

unknown. Three separate studies suggest that among young people the use of LSD on one or more occasions occurs in no more than 1 per cent of the population. The data are so imprecise that the 1 per cent figure is only a reasonable estimate, but it is clear that the statement made by advocates of LSD use, that 15 per cent of college students use LSD, is incorrect. Indeed the author of this highly publicized statement has now retracted it publicly. A carefully controlled study of a large number of young people is needed in order to assess accurately the incidence of illicit use.

The frequency of adverse reactions to LSD among illicit users is likewise unknown. Taken licitly under medical aegis, the incidence of severe untoward reactions is thought to be less than 1 per cent. Taken in uncontrolled circumstances, the incidence is far higher. Statements that only one in ten thousand has severe psychiatric reactions are arrant nonsense. As noted above, in one hospital in New York City, 130 such patients were seen in less than a two-year period. If the one in ten thousand figure were correct, simple calculations would indicate that more than one million New Yorkers are LSD users: This is patently incorrect. Thus, no valid incidence figures can be given for either illicit use or severe adverse reactions. It is clear, however, that too many people take LSD under uncontrolled circumstances, and a substantial number of these have psychotic reactions which necessitate institutionalization.

The dangers of LSD have been succinctly summarized by Dr. Sidney Cohen, a world-recognized authority on the drug. Said Dr. Cohen: "Some of the young in mind who obtain the blackmarket material will casually take it under dubious conditions and without the necessary controls. Sooner or later they will find themselves caught in the grip of pure horror. With LSD the kicks can go both ways."

This potent drug must then be reserved to the aegis of the physician for use under carefully controlled conditions. What then can be done to reduce illicit use?

The supply must be rigidly limited. At present federal law provides small incarceration penalties for unauthorized manufacture or sale. These penalties could be, and I believe should be, substantially increased, and similar laws should be passed by the individual states.

There should be both federal and state laws providing penalties for illicit possession. The dangers of illicit use are so enormous, and the benefits so nebulous, that there is no reason to condone the hedonism that engenders the indiscriminate use of LSD. There is no evidence that making unauthorized possession of LSD a misdemeanor would increase the drive to obtain black market material; rather it is likely to cause many, who would try LSD, to seek their "kicks" in some other, hopefully, potentially less dangerous fashion.

It is necessary to proscribe unauthorized manufacture, sale, or possession of any of the immediate precursors of LSD. Contrary to generally held opinion, LSD is very difficult to synthesize unless the immediate precursors are available. These include lysergic acid and its derivatives, ergotamine and ergonovine. Reduce the supply of these and the illicit manufacture of LSD will ineluctably diminish.

It is imperative to initiate a vigorous and impeccably honest campaign illustrating the potential dangers of uncontrolled LSD use. For the most part, such education at the high school and college levels is being carried out by administrators, teachers, and health officials whose knowledge about psychedelics in general and LSD in particular is frequently fragmentary, inaccurate, and often far less comprehensive than a majority of the audience they intend to convince. In any large audience there are likely to be some who would use LSD regardless of the validity of warnings against illicit use, and there will be some who under no conditions would be inveigled into illicit use. Educational movies, lectures, and discussions are then directed primarily at the large and definitely educable group who are uncommitted and often confused. If we can but provide them with facts, presented in scrupu-

lously honest fashion, the number of young individuals susceptible to the blandishments of the proselytizers should decrease.

We must, by request, cajolery, and if necessary by outright
demand, convince the communications media that they must
present the story of LSD and other psychedelics fairly and in
perspective. A heavy responsibility for the increase in illicit use
can be laid directly at their door, and no facile rationalization can
exculpate them from considerable blame for the current LSD
problem. The public has been inundated by written articles as
well as radio and television shows that, in essence, extol LSD's
virtues, trumpet its alleged ecstasies and benefits, advertise its
hedonistic qualities, and almost deliberately minimize its dangers.
A responsible press could help enormously in limiting the problem, merely by presenting a carefully balanced account, which
gives equal weight to both the horrors and joys of LSD use.

It is important that we react vigorously and continuously to the
proponents and proselytizers who would turn our already complex society into a chaotic psychedelic orgy. But we must not
overreact. Legal covenants have been suggested, for example,
which would make sale of LSD or even giving it away free a
felony punishable by a mandatory seven-year minimum sentence.
This would be unequivocal overreaction. Reasonable legal restrictions, vigorous education, and rigorous reduction of supply
should serve to limit the ravages of this hallucinogenic fad.

LSD is likely to be only the beginning. In the psychedelic
wings are bufotenine, psilocybin, mescaline, and dimethyltrypta-
mine (DMT), all of which in appropriate dosage rival the hallucinogenic capacities of LSD. Of these, the next fad is likely to
be DMT, because it is the easiest to produce chemically. We
must be prepared to cope with each of these in similar fashion to
LSD. There seems to be no evidence that the use of minor hallucinogens, such as morning glory seeds or nutmeg, will achieve
either numerical or medical significance. Their relative lack of
potency and the unpleasant side effects will likely relegate their
use for the most part to occasional experimenters or to that

coterie of social misfits whose lives are literally dedicated to psychedelics. Glue sniffing, despite the publicity surrounding it, is primarily a minor kick for the very young, usually but not always in economically deprived areas. For the most part it does not result in physical deterioration, but there are occasional reports of mental derangement and severe accidents consequent to its use, and one documented case in which glue-sniffing induced fatal bone marrow depression.

The hallucinogen most likely to defy the law and the educators is marihuana (cannabis). The literature on cannabis is both massive and contradictory. It has been declared a dire danger, a sociologic precursor leading inevitably to heroin, a cause of criminality, and contrarywise as unequivocally safe and a boon to society. From the raft of reports, statistics, and claims, the following apparently valid conclusions can be drawn. (In the following discussion, cannabis is used as the generic term and includes weak preparations such as marihuana, kif, and bhang as well as more potent preparations such as ganga, charas, or hashish.)

1. Marihuana can produce acute panic reactions, acute psychotic breaks, and profound responses mimicking the effects of LSD. The most impressive reports in this regard were written in the 1930's, when marihuana was first considerd a major sociologic problem in the United States. Indeed, in the celebrated LaGuardia Report in 1944, nine of seventy-seven persons given marihuana experimentally experienced psychotic reactions. In view of these findings, it is surprising that the report is used so extensively to substantiate the claim that marihuana is completely harmless. Nevertheless, it must be emphasized that serious adverse reactions to marihuana occur infrequently—far less often than with LSD or other potent hallucinogens.

2. Cannabis may be associated with criminality, the best documented studies having been performed in India. There the use of bhang, a cannabis derivative similar in potency to our marihuana, was *not* associated with criminality but excessive use of the more

potent cannabis preparations, ganga and charas, was associated with criminal, often violent, behavior. In the United States isolated acts of criminality or violence have occurred under the influence of marihuana, but as used here (typically a maximum of no more than one to three cigarettes a day) there is no close correlation between use and criminal activity.

3. If marihuana were used chronically in substantial amounts (more than ten cigarettes daily), the incidence of mental derangement would almost surely increase markedly. This conclusion is inferred from the experience in Morocco where kif, which is similar in potency to our marihuana, is used extensively and to excess. In that country 23 to 26 per cent of all male admissions to certain large mental hospitals were diagnosed as suffering from kif psychosis.

4. Marihuana, or any other form of cannabis, distorts time and space perception for many persons. Consequently, an individual under the drug's influence is accident-prone and is a menace behind the wheel of an auto or as the pilot of an airplane.

5. Marihuana does not inevitably lead the user to experiment with addicting drugs such as heroin. The overwhelming majority of those who use cannabis never turn to heroin, morphine, or cocaine.

6. Marihuana, at least as smoked in the United States, causes neither addiction nor physical deterioration.

It thus appears that marihuana is a mild hallucinogen which can produce acute mental derangement and if chronically used to excess may induce psychosis and/or overt antisocial behavior. The number of marihuana users in the United States is unknown, but almost surely they number in the hundreds of thousands. It is estimated that on the average, 15 per cent of college students have one or more experiences with the drug during their college career. The majority of those who do experiment with marihuana do so on only one to three occasions. Even among chronic users in the United States, the average consumption rarely exceeds a few cigarettes a day.

The arguments for legalization of marihuana are based on pure hedonism—the proponents want the legal right to use the drug because it gives them pleasure. However, the potential dangers to other persons from those who drive under the influence of marihuana, and the real possibility that legalization would create a coterie of inordinately heavy smokers, mandate the continued proscription of marihuana. Additionally, it would be hard to prevent use of the stronger, more potent forms of cannabis, which carry higher risks of psychosis and criminality. Faced with the data on potential dangers of unrestricted use of marihuana, the proponents almost uniformly rely on the argument that marihuana is no more dangerous than alcohol and therefore should be equally condoned. There are five million severe alcoholics in the United States, and more than half the serious automobile accidents are alcohol-related. Surely it would be incongruous to argue that marihuana is no worse than alcohol and should be legalized even if the addition of a large number of marihuana inebriates to the already large number of persons inebriated by alcohol might mean a profound increase in the incidence of lethal automobile accidents. Obviously the major criterion for any drug should not be a comparison with already legalized alcohol but rather the inherent dangers in indiscriminate use of that drug. If this criterion were not rigidly adhered to, there would be a proliferation of drugs dispensed merely for pleasure, and if each of these carried risks of physical and/or mental harm similar to alcohol and cigarettes, then the number of persons damaged by the pleasure-producing drugs would inevitably increase strikingly. Surely society has a right, indeed an obligation to limit the distribution of potentially dangerous and medically useless drugs.

If use of nonmedicinal drugs is to be restricted, it is imperative that care be taken to exempt necessary escape mechanisms (such as alcohol appears to be for our society) and to enforce drug interdictions with just—but not cruel—penalties. There can be no quarrel with the rather harsh covenants covering illicit sale or smuggling of cannabis. It is, however, an unfortunate fact that the federal government and the majority of individual states continue in anachronistic fashion to treat identically the user of marihuana and the user of far more dangerous drugs such as heroin. Recently the federal law has been modified so that marihuana use is treated slightly less stringently, but this is a small and pusillanimous step. What is needed is complete recodification of our dangerous drug laws to remove marihuana from its legal heroin embrace and place it in the entirely separate category of hallucinogens. In this regard it is interesting to note that at present, possession of thirty marihuana cigarettes is a felony in New York State, and at the federal level conviction on a charge of marihuana possession incurs a two-year penalty. Yet possession of an ounce of pure LSD, a far more potent hallucinogen, is only a misdemeanor in New York State and is no crime at all at the federal level. These nonsensical inconsistencies can be set right only by total revamping of our narcotic-hallucinogen laws.

If recodification were carried out, it would permit changes in the laws regarding marihuana possession. Clearly these are currently far too harsh. Mere possession has sometimes resulted in sentences of between one and fifteen years. Reducing the penalty for the user of marihuana should in no way impair vigorous attack on the venal smugglers, importers, and sellers of cannabis preparations.

As with LSD, the most effective attack on illicit marihuana use is continuous, honest, and vigorous education, including a frank admission that marihuana as used in America is, for the non-driver, far less dangerous than LSD or DMT or even hashish. Specious statements concerning physical deterioration due to marihuana or inexorable progression to heroin can only serve to negate otherwise valid educational efforts.

There is an additional problem which merits discussion. The increasing use of psychedelic drugs is only one consequence of a profound liberalization of the moral code in America. In a society that has adopted an almost insouciant attitude toward sexual and public morality, permissiveness in regard to use of many drugs, including psychedelics, has become commonplace. Extension of permissiveness to drug use creates direct conflicts with our laws. Permissiveness cannot be equated with illegality; yet this is exactly what our younger people are doing, abetted by many older persons including educators. Premarital sexual promiscuity is often condoned by a society in which moral guidelines have been relaxed; but use of marihuana, and in some states potent hallucinogens such as LSD, falls under the aegis not of moral and social guidelines but of our established legal codes. Unmarried persons of adult age who experiment with sex may be accused of immorality, but those who use drugs such as marihuana are criminals.

Articulating the differences between permissiveness and illegality and urging young persons to obey our laws is considered by many to be a waste of time. It is my belief, however, that this undramatic and unexciting approach to drug abuse is, together with the arguments advanced above concerning the dangers, absolutely necessary. And although it is likely to be greeted with derision and haughty rejection by young persons, it is fundamentally a sound and persuasive argument. If a promarihuana group can with impunity flaunt the marihuana laws, and pro-LSD groups ignore the LSD laws, then any group with a given vested interest can defy and violate any law. Such actions lead inevitably to moral and legal chaos. If one believes, as I do, that we are basically a land of law-abiding citizens, then attractively packaged arguments that urge compliance with our existing laws or modification of them by traditional democratic techniques fall for the most part on receptive ears, even if identification with their peer group compels young listeners to outwardly reject such concepts as anachronistic.

It seems clear that the use of psychedelic drugs for hedonistic purposes will remain a problem during the coming years. A careful blending of flexibility, exhortation, education, laws, limitation of supply, and rehabilitative efforts should permit us to minimize the numbers of persons involved and retain the overwhelming majority of our young people as productive, active members of society.

In the United States approximately 12,000 kilograms of potent opiates were administered for legitimate purposes in 1962 according to a United Nations survey. Additionally, some 60,000 to 120,000 persons habitually use opiates illicitly every year. Over 90 per cent of those addicted use diacetylmorphine (heroin); the others take dilaudid, methadone, morphine, opium, codeine, or demerol. For the most part abusers of these drugs reside in areas of blight in large cities. Indeed, almost 80 per cent of the known narcotics addicts in the United States live in ten large municipalities, more than half of these in either New York City or Chicago. Recent reports have emphasized the spread of this problem into suburban communities, but the fact remains that the Negro, Puerto Rican, and Mexican ghettoes of our cities spawn most of the country's addiction; 70 per cent of all addicts belong to one of these three ethnic groups. Most addicts are under thirty years of age. In this brief account I should like to discuss some of the myths of drug addiction, what motivates young persons to turn to heroin, the major complications, past treatment programs, the approach in Great Britain, and the most hopeful programs being undertaken in the United States.

SOME MYTHS

Addicts are violent persons given to mugging and homicide. The data clearly show this statement is specious. In point of fact, addicts commit an inordinate number of crimes against property —burglary, forgery, stealing, but they show no greater tendency than the general public to commit aggravated assault. In some areas heroin users commit homicide more often than the general population, but most of their violence is directed against pushers or other drug users, not against innocent bystanders. Addicts may indeed commit violence during a criminal spree to obtain money for drugs, but this is unusual and the heroin user will generally avoid such offenses if possible.

Addicts frequently commit sex crimes. This is arrant nonsense. Heroin reduces sexual desire. There is not one whit of evidence that rape or other sexual crimes can be related to opiate abuse.

The heroin seller (pusher) seeks out new converts. Addiction is contagious in the sense that addicts create new addicts, but the concept of a pusher loitering around a school waiting for innocent children is spurious. The heroin user seeks out the pusher, who is a venal but passive parasite.

One shot of heroin inevitably leads to addiction. Actually some persons use heroin intermittently without ever becoming addicted. Among those who do become physically addicted, the duration from first injection to physical dependence ranges from two weeks to one year.

Once a person becomes habituated to several injections of heroin daily, abrupt discontinuation of the drug results in severe, even violent symptoms, including nausea, vomiting, abdominal pain, chills, and fever. In point of fact, the heroin is usually adulterated (cut) so extensively that physical addiction occurs relatively infrequently. Consequently, most heroin users taking one to six injections (costing $5-30 daily) can be readily withdrawn with either small amounts of barbiturates or tranquilizers or no medicaments at all. Those using larger amounts or obtaining less adulterated heroin must be withdrawn slowly, usually with methadone or a similar narcotic as a substitute. Currently the major difficulties in withdrawal relate not to addiction to heroin but rather to mixed heroin-barbiturate addiction, since abrupt withdrawal from barbiturates in a barbiturate addict may produce high fever, convulsions, and even death.

Marihuana use leads to abuse of opiates. There is no evidence that marihuana per se leads to heroin. The majority of heroin users first used marihuana, but contrariwise, the overwhelming majority of the estimated 200,000,000 persons in the world who use marihuana or similar substances never progress to heroin use. In the United States 15 per cent of college students are said to use marihuana one or more times, yet virtually none of these subsequently turns to heroin.

Heroin addiction is a chronic, incurable disease. There are large numbers of addicts who, after age thirty to thirty-five and for reasons that are not clear, no longer need the crutch of heroin and discontinue use on their own. This self-discontinuation of opiates has been termed the maturing out process. The fact that addicts can and do cure themselves indicates that if the appropriate techniques are found, young addicts can indeed be cured.

REASONS FOR STARTING HEROIN

In middle-class neighborhoods heroin is used infrequently. Here the individual starts using it because in his particular community there is a drug-oriented peer group (often small in numbers), in which heroin use is already rampant. Many of these middle and upper-class youngsters have substantial psychiatric abnormalities.

The story is somewhat different in the slum areas. Here, in certain localities, heroin abuse is much more frequent. Use of heroin results from a combination of environmental deprivations, family disunity, personality defects, and peer group use. In these areas of urban blight, prejudice, undereducation, lack of job opportunity, poverty, and inadequate housing combine to make a milieu which creates frustration and an urge for rebellion. Additionally, Chein has found that many heroin users come from broken homes characterized by loss of a father figure. The user himself tends to be immature, self-centered, non-goal-directed, and incapable of tolerating frustration. The environment, family breakdown, and defective personality act in concert to make the individual susceptible to drug abuse. His rebellion against society results in drug use in large part because of the ready availability of heroin in these blighted areas and because many of his peer group are using the drug. In an attempt to belong, to avoid being called scared, as a sign of anger against the affluent society he feels he cannot join, or merely as a lark at a party, the susceptible individual tries heroin and then, driven by his personality defects, becomes habituated (defined as chronic use) or addicted (defined as physical dependence).

THE COMPLICATIONS—SOCIOLOGICAL AND MEDICAL

The habitué or addict soon becomes entirely isolated. His whole life revolves around drug use and his circle of acquaintances and friends shrinks to exclude all but those who are heroin users. As drug use continues, the addict usually turns to crime to obtain funds for the heroin, rejects regular employment, and becomes a pariah, isolated from the society against which he has rebelled. The men not infrequently turn to selling heroin (80 per cent of street sellers are themselves heroin users), and the women to prostitution. In New York City, for example, the majority of arrested street-walking prostitutes are heroin users, plying their trade to get money for the drug.

Thus the heroin addict becomes ensnared in a vicious cycle, which leads ineluctably to depravity, degradation, and despair. Additionally, he subjects himself to a variety of potentially severe medical complications. The most serious of these is overdose. This occurs when the user injects himself with too large a dose of heroin. It may occur immediately after he has been incarcerated, or when, on returning to the community, he injects himself with his preincarceration dose, which is now too strong for a body that no longer is acclimated to heroin. More often it happens because the user has no idea what he is injecting—the concentration of heroin in street packets has been shown to range from 0 to 77 per cent. .

Once overdose has occurred, the user becomes stuporous and in severe cases, comatose; death may then supervene. One per cent (200-300) of all addicts in New York City die of overdoses every year. This is a staggering figure since it is a measure of one of the major areas of death among young, otherwise healthy, people in New York City.

A second severe medical complication is hepatitis, a viral infection of the liver, in this case transmitted by unsterile needles. Although often requiring hospitalization for weeks or even months, hepatitis is not usually fatal. It can, however, lead to permanent liver damage and on occasion can be lethal. Recent studies suggest that 75 per cent of chronic heroin users suffer from hepatitis, and at Bellevue Hospital in New York City 55 per cent of all cases of hepatitis are related to heroin use.

Other medical complications include endocarditis (a frequently fatal infection of the heart valves) and tetanus. The latter, which carries a mortality of over 50 per cent, occurs primarily in older addicts who have scarred their veins and then have resorted to subcutaneous injection of heroin (skin popping). The heroin and its adulterants are irritating, and the ensuing inflammation provides an ideal nidus for growth of the bacterium that causes tetanus.

Addicts are also susceptible to a variety of skin infections and to inflammation of the veins into which heroin is injected.

PAST ATTEMPTS AT REHABILITATION

As noted above, it is important to recognize that if the addict lives to age thirty-five, he is likely to discontinue heroin use on his own. Consequently, to be considered effective, rehabilitation programs must reach the addict in his teens and early twenties. In the past, most programs have been abysmal failures. The relapse rate after discharge from the Public Health Service facility at Lexington, Kentucky, was 95 per cent, although the five-year follow-up of the same population of discharges showed a voluntary abstinence rate of 25 per cent. A follow-up study of patients discharged from the Riverside Hospital in New York City indicated that almost all promptly returned to heroin abuse.

Three studies merit emphasis, for each suggests that the key to success is well-supervised after-care. The New York State Division of Parole followed approximately six hundred jailed addicts in a parole program with a high case worker to parolee ratio. Approximately one-third of these ill-motivated heroin users made a satisfactory adjustment, defined as a return to the community, employment, and freedom from drug abuse. Virtually identical results were obtained in a similar number of patients studied by the New York City Parole Commission. Vaillant followed patients discharged from the Lexington facility and found a greater abstinence rate among those supervised under parole programs than among voluntary admissions who had no such after-care supervision.

These three studies form the basis for the concept that no inpatient program can succeed unless accompanied by rigorous supervision for a substantial period of time after discharge.

THE BRITISH SYSTEM

In England an addict has been permitted to obtain heroin on prescription. No attempts at rehabilitation have been mandated, and for the most part, the heroin users do not work steadily, instead congregating in pubs and gradually increasing membership in their drug subculture. In the last five years, the number of addicts has doubled, and if youthful heroin users are considered separately, a six-fold increase has occurred. The incidence of opiate addiction in Great Britain is now estimated at four to five per 100,000. This is far smaller than the fifty to sixty per 100,000 estimated for the United States, but the increment in incidence in the United Kingdom is far greater than in the United States, where the number of habitués and addicts has remained virtually stationary for the last ten years.

The rapid increase in illicit heroin use and resulting addiction has alarmed British authorities. It seems likely that restrictions will be placed on pharmacists and physicians. Whether this will curb Britain's burgeoning problem is problematical unless attempts are made to reduce the illicit supply and rehabilitate established addicts.

CURRENT REHABILITATION PROGRAMS OF PROMISE IN THE UNITED STATES

Civil commitment. New York State and California have initiated civil commitment programs in which arrested addicts are sent to rehabilitation facilities rather than jail. Nonarrested heroin users can also apply for voluntary admission. Additionally, nonarrested addicts can be involuntarily committed, in New York for up to three years, in California for up to seven years. This latter provision has stimulated vitriolic debate, but the polemics appear unwarranted, since both states appear to be reserving such commitment for a small number of individuals referred by close relatives. The California program is centered in a massive single rehabilitation unit in which group therapy is the mainstay of treatment. After-care is rigorously supervised by parole officers. Initial results show that two and one-half years after discharge the recovery rate is a discouraging 12 per cent, but the rigid criteria for recovery may make this figure deceptively low. New York State's superbly funded program was started in April 1967: It is obviously too early to make any predictions concerning success, but this does stand as the most ambitious rehabilitative effort ever undertaken for narcotic addicts.

Rehabilitation without drugs (other than the civil commitment programs). A variety of voluntary and governmental agencies are attempting to treat small numbers of addicts with counseling, individual psychotherapy, or general supportive measures. Additionally, three groups have initiated large-scale rehabilitative efforts based primarily on group therapy. These include Synanon,

Daytop, and the Ramirez program in New York City. Synanon has treated over fifteen hundred, approximately half of whom have not completed the prescribed therapy period. Of the rest, only a handful have been returned to the community. The Synanon program consists of in-patient group living in an inordinately rigid environment in which the individual is subjugated to the group and undergoes abrasive ego destruction before attempts at rebuilding and personality are made. The cult-like existence of Synanon, its refusal to accept extramural evaluation, and its disinclination to return addicts to the community limit its value as a treatment program, although it is clear that this type of experience is beneficial for a small number of well-motivated addicts.

Daytop is a Synanon offshoot which utilizes group therapy, often conducted primarily by ex-addicts, and frequently direct and abrasive. Unlike Synanon, the Daytop group-living program is open to impartial evaluation, accepts initially ill-motivated addicts, and after a period of one to two years returns the individual to the community. Although preliminary reports are optimistic, this approach needs the test of time and careful extramural scrutiny.

The Ramirez approach is likewise in its inchoate phases. It consists of three parts. During an out-patient community-based phase, attempts are made to inculcate motivation in the addict. This part of the program is conducted almost exclusively by ex-addicts. The second phase consists of one and one-half to two years of hospitalization, during which various types of group therapy are employed. For the third phase of the treatment schedule the addict is followed closely back in the community, first in a halfway house and then fully on his own. Whether the encouraging results obtained in Puerto Rico can be repeated in the heroin center of the Western world, New York City, remains to be seen.

Rehabilitation with drugs. The two drugs currently used are methadone, an addicting opiate, and cyclazocine, a synthetic drug, chemically related to morphine, which acts as a narcotic antagonist. The best known methadone program is being conducted in New York City under the supervision of Drs. Vincent Dole and Marie Nyswander. Addicts must be volunteers and are generally rejected if they manifest mixed addictions. Those accepted after a careful screening procedure are stabilized on methadone, which keeps them addicted but prevents them from feeling the effects of heroin. Thus they can take methadone once daily and spend the day in school, at work, or in other activities of the extensive rehabilitative panoply which is an essential part of the program. Only six weeks are spent in the hospital, the methadone being dispensed on an out-patient basis thereafter.

Preliminary results are indeed very encouraging, but it is important to stress certain caveats—the patients are well motivated, they remain addicted, many are rejected during the screening process, and the adscititious rehabilitative efforts are extensive. At present this is an important experiment, but it is clearly not yet suitable for the addict population in general, nor is it clear whether the good results are in any way related to the methadone. It will indeed be interesting to see what happens when the methadone is withdrawn and when the program is expanded to include less-well-motivated, unselected addicts.

The studies on cyclazocine are so limited as to make even preliminary interpretation impossible. This drug prevents an opiate from having any effect and is not significantly addicting. It does, however, have its own moderately annoying, but not incapacitating, side effects. Whether it can be used, combined with other rehabilitative efforts, to treat heroin addiction effectively remains to be seen.

In summary, heroin addiction remains a persistent sociological malignancy in the United States. Its prevalence has changed little over the last decade, but it has defied efforts to diminish or eradicate it. At present vigorous attempts are being made through a variety of experimental programs to rehabilitate the established addict. Surely some of these will be at least moderately effective.

But the scourge of opiate abuse will not be eliminated or even profoundly reduced until efforts at rehabilitation are equally matched by more vigorous law enforcement directed against importers, distributors, and street pushers, and by extensive preventive education in endemic areas. Above all, we as a society must fully commit ourselves to eradicate urban blight, for it is in the slums that heroin addiction has its genesis: abolish them, and inevitably much of the heroin abuse will disappear.

NOTE ON CONTRIBUTOR

Donald B. Louria (M.D., 1953, Harvard Medical School) is head of the infectious diseases laboratory and is visiting physician at Bellevue Hospital, New York City. He also is associate professor of medicine, Cornell University Medical College, New York. He prepared position papers on medicine and public health for John Lindsay, present mayor of New York City, during his campaign for office. Governor of New York Nelson Rockefeller named Dr. Louria to head a council on drug addiction for the state. He currently serves on the Committee on Problems of Drug Dependence, National Research Council, National Academy of Science, Division of Medicine Sciences.

3

Contraceptive Methods for Global Control of Population

JOHN ROCK, M.D.

TODAY, AT LONG LAST, one is not called upon to fight for theoretical approval of birth control. Throughout the civilized world the battle for the minds of intelligent people on that particular issue has been won. Winning acceptance of the theory, however, was but the first battle in the war for the integrity of human society, indeed for the future welfare of our species. The war is still being waged. There is a wide gap between theory and practice. The validity of the theory must so impress all peoples as to energize them to act upon it.

What is meant by "integrity of society"? Integrity is defined as "an unimpaired condition"; and society as "an enduring, cooperating social group so functioning as to maintain itself and perpetuate the species." The social units that must individually endure and cooperate, each with all others, so that human society will maintain itself and perpetuate the species, are the individual families. During the last decade sociologists have reached general agreement that in every human society, all over the globe, the characteristic family structure is that of monogamy: the man and the woman, in an approved union, and their offspring. The universality of this unit grouping, I believe, attests to its biological origin: Better than by any other structuring, monogamous marriage facilitates expression of man's inherent sex-instinct, characteristically suffused, as it is, with enduring love of mate and of offspring. For full response to this humanly embellished instinct, mankind instituted, and throughout the ages has maintained the monogamous family pattern. Within this design, up to the present, man has perpetuated the species. There now appear grave reasons to fear that this will not remain possible for long, unless he manifests the wisdom that justifies his species designation as Homo *sapiens*. Easily, as he has well demonstrated, he can continue to propagate; but can he surely continue to reproduce healthy, adult human beings?

Our species is unique among all animals: It, only, is endowed with intellectuality. Our properly fed animal body grows, and in mating, procreates automatically. But our intellects utterly require education and correcty apperceived experience; and apperception utterly requires correlation of what is experienced with previously acquired knowledge. To ensure perpetuation of our species, then, parents themselves must have knowledge and must make certain its transmission to their offspring. So intricate has our evolved culture become that parents—together with their surrogates, other teachers—can do this only if the number of offspring within the whole group of families is limited to parental and institutional capabilities.

Statistics clearly show that, at least for the time being, developed nations, including the United States, have reached this limit. And they show even more clearly that in the underdeveloped nations three-quarters of humanity has already exceeded the limit. For mankind in general, to transform easily achieved parentage into species-required parenthood, global birth rates must be controlled; indeed, in most of the world, greatly restricted.

I must interpolate a warning to us of the United States who are perhaps too smug. As long ago as 1961 Dr. Donald Bogue, Professor of Sociology at the University of Chicago, said what is still true: "The United States is faced with a population problem that is as acute as any in Asia or Africa or Latin America." He meant that our over-all standard of living is in as much jeopardy from our growth rate as are the base levels in many other areas.

I think it appropriate also to call to the attention of wishful thinkers that any proposed or already achieved increase of food production will be useless for social salvation. Like all of us, these dear people are well aware that world food production is at present far less than meets human capabilities. Furthermore, our present technical ability to extend our efforts has hardly begun to utilize many new sources of food, oceanic and synthetic for instance. Admittedly, agricultural science alone promises vast augmentation of terrestrial yields. In time there can be food aplenty for many, many more mouths than now need it. But man's fecundity will not of itself lie fallow during the time required to achieve this increase. Permit me to quote the trenchant words of Lamont C. Cole, Professor of Zoology at Cornell University:

The growth of any population, plant or animal, can be resolved. . . . qualitatively into two phenomena, the capacity of the organisms to increase in numbers and the capacity of the environment to support organisms of that type. All species are potentially capable of increase beyond the capacity of the environment. The earth, or for that matter, the universe, is not large enough to contain all the house-flies, or mushrooms that would exist after a few generations if the potential rate of increase could be sustained. The same generalization applies to elephants, whales, men, and sequoia trees; they would simply take a little longer to fill the universe . . .

I propose that we all now assume responsibility for the essential requirement: The fecundity of human beings must be restrained. The most advanced groups, in the already developed countries, who enjoy and profit by the highest standards of living, should realize this beyond question. We now know that the security of the monogamous family, which I believe is the naturally evolved structural unit of society the world over, utterly depends on full expression of intrafamilial love combined with strict conscientious limitation of biological parentage. Clearly the continued evolutionary convergence of human society demands not parentage, but good parenthood; not procreation, but reproduction of mature, healthy, reasoning adults. This is best accomplished within the close-knit family soundly constructed by intelligent, loving parents, who know how mutually to enjoy and to profit from their sexuality, while they fully express their species responsibilities.

I repeat, for the benefit of the pitiable "ostriches," that the first battle in the war for social safety has been won: There is consensus among informed men and women that worldwide responsible parenthood is an unavoidable obligation. I direct your attention to the statement of Dr. Philip Hauser, the distinguished sociologist: "It is possible to state at the present time that there are no value systems, including religious value systems, that are opposed to responsible parenthood." I would add: There is every evidence that the vast majority of intelligent people the world over now realize that good parenthood for all peoples cannot be accomplished without the restriction of fecundity which we call "birth control." Yet this kind of parenthood is approaching impossibility in the hopefully called "developing" nations of Central and South America, of Africa and Southeast Asia, in which areas live three-quarters of humankind. It is clearly not possible among them for parents in general to exercise socially constructive, educational, and health-conditioning parenthood.

Global growth rates must be cut. Repeatedly it has been emphasized that growth rates are but the difference between birth rates and death rates. Our inescapable humanitarianism forbids increasing the latter. Indeed, it demands quite the contrary. All over the world we struggle to eradicate disease. We bend every effort to fight death. Hence it is the birth rates that must be cut radically and promptly. But how? This is the battle we now must fight successfully if we are to win the war for the security of mankind.

Let us examine our arsenal. What weapons have we? How can

they best be used? In what way can we improve them and facilitate their adequate use?

The United Nations Advisory Mission on Family Planning in India expertly evaluated the best of our present armamentarium as it could function in India if each method were efficiently used. I refer to their appraisal of present methods as they relate to India only because of the high quality of the Mission's study and because the vicious situation in India so clearly manifests what already threatens all the developing nations in South America, Southeast Asia, and Africa. In these areas about three-quarters of all human beings on earth are now struggling against rapidly approaching disaster. The most competent demographers and agriculturists have demonstrated the utter impossibility of continually increasing world food production fast enough to catch up, much less to keep up with the needs of our accelerating growth-rates.

In India, where *each year* the population already increases by more than ten million, the United Nations Mission reckoned that raising the age of marriage would in one decade reduce this growth by at least 10 per cent.

Throughout mankind, monogamous marriage has evolved as the best structure for human sexuality if this is to serve its primary biological purpose: species survival, *i.e.,* preservation of uniquely spiritual humanity. Physical sexual development in the growing boy and girl is automatic and reaches powerful mating-proclivity by midadolescence. Parenthood that fulfills its responsibility will firmly equip each boy and girl with what is indispensable for the subjugation of this physical copulatory urge to the welfare of society. *Pari passu* with its development, there must be clear understanding of the physical, and particularly the mental dynamics of human sex-functioning. To this insight there must be added willing submission to rationally accepted, pertinent, and potent social sanctions, which are but the constantly improving distillates of our evolving humanity.

Sex education of this sort is essential if marriage is to be long withheld without impulsive self-debasement of youths, by their exploitation of maidens, themselves not altogether guiltless. Though through the centuries in more advanced cultures some progress has been made here and there in checking expression of sexual maturation until slower growing intellectuality justifies it, the potentially good method of later marriage cannot be expected to bring prompt reduction of birth rates in the developing countries. Nevertheless it should be worked on, just as we in the United States must oppose any approach to parentage by those incapable of direct or indirect good parenthood.

The United Nations Mission figured that sterilization of either husband or wife of a mating that had completed its social obligation in numbers of healthy children would, in one decade, cut India's annual growth by about 20 per cent.

The essential requirement for restriction of births among all nations, rich and poor, is prevention of access of male and female germ cells to one another. This can be achieved by suppression of production of one or the other, or by complete blockage of the avenue of their mutual approach. Sterlization means the latter. Sterlization of the wife, in this context, requires only a simple minor surgical procedure that interrupts the tubal pathway through which spermatozoa proceed to meet with the egg. If this operation is performed just after a delivery, it need not increase or prolong the mother's disability. Because it requires entering the pelvic cavity, usually through a small abdominal incision, if done at other times, a short few days of hospitalization are mandatory. Of course such tubal surgery has no effect on other aspects of reproductive functioning: Menstruation and feminine qualities are not changed. Infertility is immediate.

To confine the husband's sperm is even simpler. This requires only interruption in the patency of the tiny duct on each side of the scrotum through which germ cells pass from the testicles into the upper portion of the urinary passage. This entails only a small incision through the scrotum or of the groin on each side. Bed rest is not always necessary and discomfort is minimal. Because there remain masses of spermatozoa in the portions of the ducts between the interruption and the penis, this procedure is contraceptively unreliable for at least four weeks.

Until not much more than one hundred years ago moralists were unavoidably ignorant of the nature and function of both male and female germ cells. This lack of knowledge led to what now appears fantastic speculation, which attributed high esteem to these only potentially useful cells. However, while this concept prevailed, sterilization was held to be at least thoroughly reprehensible. One contributory misconception was that these germ cells, which in themselves are not wholly human, were nevertheless entitled to the dignity and respect due living, completely human parts.

For a long time it has been known that these short-lived organisms, both male and female, lack one-half of the characterizing, species-designating chromosomes. Not until they unite is there a human cell present. This is conception; and the conceived unit has become human and must, from then on, be treated as such. Nature discards or destroys all but a tiny proportion of the single male and female germ cells that are produced. Uncomplemented by one of the opposite sex, these individual cells are actually useless to both their makers and society. Only when the one from one mate combines with the one from the other mate comes the actuality that is essential for species preservation. Before their recognition, only about a century and a half ago, the preciousness of the few that do combine bestowed on all an unwarrantedly exalted respect. Furthermore, in their physiological ignorance people became accustomed to equating the potentiality of germ cells with sexual capability—with virile manhood and thorough femaleness. Nor could they realize the culpable lack of charity in procreation that cannot ensure reproduction of a healthy rational adult.

The reordering of the evaluation of uncomplemented germ cells requires a degree of insight and psychological adjustment that comes hard for uneducated people. Perhaps this is just as well for the happiness of many parents. Immediate conditions that might make sterilization attractive, notably enough children and their drain on parental resources, may change and render some of these germ cells again desirable for both the family and society. Success in re-establishment of their availability, by further surgery to open again the ducts that have been occluded, is still of only moderate possibility, yet of certain inconvenience and expense as well as of slight hazard, especially in the female. Because of these very real objections—practical, psychological, cultural (mostly religious), and because of the surgery and expense involved, this theoretically excellent method of birth control is not likely to effect, in the immediate future, the imminently required decrease in the birth rates of most countries.

Surprisingly, however, in sorely distressed India, wherever adequate social and medical facilities were well organized and properly proffered, sterilization has met with wide acceptance. In our own country, with superior obstetrical and urological facilities, innumerable perspicacious or only madly harassed parents of as many or more children as could be constructively cared for have gladly accepted this basically harmless solution. It is surprising to many among us how gradually more and more of our educated people are choosing this way to secure family stability and the prospect of a happy, useful life for their children. However, because family tragedies do occur, surgical escape may bring subsequent grim regrets for wives under forty and husbands under fifty. It is also, I think, inadvisable for all who are not psychologically quite stable and well informed. It has been reliably estimated that during the late 1950's 45,000 American husbands and 65,000 American wives willingly had recourse to sterilization, and the number is steadily increasing. In India, during the seven years preceding 1964, this method was chosen by 250,000 men and 150,000 women. Its acceptability among intelligent but uneducated peoples is not to be underestimated. Its simplicity, with completeness and finality of relief from worry by a single decision, renders it attractive in areas where facilities are available.

The vexing requirements of astute social services and thoroughly capable surgical personnel and adequate equipment do not make sterilization unworthy of at least thoughtful consideration as a contributory solution to the urgency of reducing birth rates in those of the developing countries that are fortunately free of cultural overvaluation of half-human germ cells.

The worrisome urgency of relief from excessive numbers, and the fact that the prospect of ruinous famine has rapidly overtaken us while older methods of birth control have been well known must not blind us to the continuing practical efficacy of some of them now, when the need is greatest. The condom, for instance, has doubtless been of great assistance to several generations, but notably only among peoples of high motivation—which is largely proportionate to literacy. In overpopulous areas of underdeveloped countries, educational facilities are meager, and motivation to reach worthy but dimly detected goals is weak at best. The requirements of antecedent provision of contraceptive articles or substances for immediate use render them only moderately helpful where illiteracy is high and birth rates are most threatening or already disastrous.

In India, nevertheless, proposed furtherance of use of the condom could diminish the growth rate by the not inconsiderable amount of 10 per cent in the judgment of the United Nations Commission. In Latin America and Africa this desirable result from the condom seems very unlikely. Cultural attitudes in these areas still maintain the primitive misconception that a man's fecundity is evidence of his prestigious manhood. To limit the family is selfishly thought to be woman's business.

Raising the age of marriage, sterilization, and use of the condom, all efficacious measures if widely achieved, are severely handicapped where needed most. This is not mainly because distress from large families is not realized, but largely because illiteracy has kept the people ignorant of the fact that children need not be spawned, themselves to live lives of misery.

Anent this, Alberto Lleras Comargo, former President of the Republic of Colombia, South America, wrote in 1964:

> The root cause for continuing high birth rates in Latin America is the nearly total ignorance of birth control on the part of the masses rather than any organized resistance to it. Studies in Puerto Rico, Peru, Chile and Mexico generally show the lower classes to be over-whelmingly in favor of small families and receptive toward birth control. But about the only contraceptive technique they know is sexual abstention. For obvious reasons this method wins no popularity contests.

The time and personnel required to indoctrinate use of these methods force us to utilize and to offer our less-favored global neighbors other more immediately promising contraceptive measures.

Prominent among these is the so-called "pill." In my discussion I use the designation *pill* in a generic sense, to mean any of the preparations containing both female sex hormones in one tablet. There are some ten different preparations of such oral medicines already approved by our Federal Food and Drug Administration. If properly used, they prevent ovulation. Tablets containing less than 2 mg. of combined hormones are not to be trusted, however, during the first cycle of treatment. The unique advantage of the pill is that it prevents release of an egg by the same hormonologic process as functions to suppress a second ovulation, during a menstrual cycle, if one egg has already been set free; as also, by essentially the same process that holds throughout the nine months of a normal pregnancy. Nature so arranges suppression of ovulation that no competing conception can occur to jeopardize the one that may be or already has been established. In nature all this is done by the woman's built-in protective mechanism. This ceases to function, though, a few weeks after the baby is born. But if the mother's brain tells her that her infant, after leaving her protective body, still needs her resources, and she responds, mentally, by willfully placing the baby at breast, the infant's nursing reactivates her hormonal suppression of further ovulation and maintains this infertility as long as suckling brings full production of milk.

By the same token, if the brain of a nonpregnant or nursing woman tells her that, were ovulation to occur, there would arise the possibility of a pregnancy that would seriously endanger her usefulness for the best parenthood of which she would be capable, and she responds by willful and proper use of the pill (again by exercise of the same intellect that re-established suppression of ovulation by placement of her infant at breast), she inhibits the potentially dangerous ovulation by essentially the same hormonologic process that functioned in the last two weeks of each menstrual cycle, month after month, as also during pregnancy and full nursing. To my mind this is, up to now, our only method of voluntary contraception that can be called a "natural method of birth control." Resentful continence within marriage, that for most people characterizes the rhythm method, to me does not appear in Nature's plan for monogamous marriage and responsible parenthood.

As with many other basically natural processes, the action of the pill has its disadvantages. When present, they appear to be quite comparable to disturbances of intrinsic hormone interplay during the postovulatory phase in each menstrual cycle, as well as during pregnancy and lactation. Compared to the effect of the body's own hormones, though, the pill-action on the body in general, exclusive of the ovary where it does no damage, is much weaker than that of the greater hormone concentrations in pregnancy.

Because of this similarity in over-all effect, there may appear any of the uncomfortable disorderings that are sometimes suffered by one woman or another during the two weeks preceding menstruation, or during pregnancy or lactation. Obviously we do not meet with those attributable to the growing occupant of the womb, or to its later activation of the breasts by nursing. Many of those well-known and rather accepted side effects are encountered now and then among patients who are using one or another of the authorized preparations. Most frequently is temporary slight nausea. Edema, *i.e.,* retention of water in body tissues notably in the lower extremities, is also not uncommon. These often accompany pregnancy. Such fluid retention may, in susceptible individuals, predispose and very occasionally lead to phlebitis, venous clotting, and even perhaps to embolism—the dispersion or migration of a blood clot. The specific culpability of the pill in these latter conditions—dramatic, possibly tragic—has not yet been proved. These vascular disturbances all occur now and then in the nonpregnant, nonmedicated woman. They are more common during pregnancy, and particularly in the period after delivery. They are even found in men.

Very occasionally, after cessation of pill medication, menstruation may be harmlessly delayed, even for some months. Vastly more common than failure to flow is prompt susceptibility to normal pregnancy, when use of the pill ceases. Women who just before menstruation or during pregnancy experience mental disturbances, such as emotional instability, depression, irritability, forgetfulness, vagueness, etc., may possibly note the same with the pill. More often, medication seems to make any that habitually occurred before menstruation less likely or less objectionable.

Much ill-advised, unsubstantiated, and unwarranted scaremongering has been indulged in by lugubrious theorists that the pill may cause cancer. Actually, the carefully gathered and analyzed statistics concerning this, after ten years of wide use of the pill, suggest quite the opposite. The same may be said of findings from careful experimentation with animals that are not characteristically prone to malignancy.

Similarly, the fear of delay of the physiological infertility of the menopause, as also of a late recurrence of fertility, are utterly irrational and have never resulted from pill medication. The eggs remaining in the ovary after long use of the pill are no more or less old and sterile in the woman of given age than they would be anyway. As for safety in duration of pill suppression of ovulation, there appears to be no more of a limit to this than there is to promptly repeated sequences of pregnancy, with or without the extension of inhibition of ovulation by lactation. To be sure, repetitions of these conditions are preceded by one to four ovulations; but this, in good theory and practice, does not destroy the similarity in effects.

If sexuality is affected, toward increase or decrease, in women who do not ordinarily show such variations during unmedicated menstrual cycles, the change, if noted, seems in almost all cases to be purely of psychological origin and not chemically related to the ingredients of the pill.

In spite of the very generally harmless, 100 per cent efficacy of proper pills used correctly, this superior method of family planning for the parents in already developed countries is as yet severely handicapped in the countries most in need of birth control. Because of the enumerated various possible side effects, pill medication everywhere requires a certain degree of medical supervision. The pill can never be a simple over-the-counter chain-store, even drug store or lay-supervised item. Medical and adequately trained paramedical personnel are hard to come by in impoverished crowded areas of countries straining hard to achieve economic stability. Furthermore, the cost of the pill is still too high to expect immediate realization of its great potentiality in decreasing distressful growth rates. Essential, also, under presently effective regimens for use of the pill, are high motivation, the ability to count calendar days, and appropriate safe places in which to keep these highly efficient species-protective preparations.

The other valuable addition to our armamentarium is the so-called intra-uterine device, the IUD. Of this there are some four or five slightly different forms. Those governmentally approved share apparent chemical innocuousness within the womb, and are comparatively inexpensive. My further remarks concerning them pertain largely to the three older and more commonly used forms: the loop, the coil, and the bow, and more specifically to the first two, the loop and the coil. These consist of short rods, about 1.5 mm. in diameter, of the inert plastic, polyethylene. The loop is molded in serpentine shape; the coil, as a spiral. The shaped rods are easily straightened so as to fit into a metal tubule specially designed for their placement in the uterine cavity. When the tubule is withdrawn and the plastic IUD left behind, this promptly resumes its manufactured form as a loop or as a coil. Thus it lies flattened between the front and back walls of the womb, pressing gently on the mucous membrane of these and against their side borders where these walls merge one into the other.

How IUD's function to prevent diagnosable pregnancy in almost all of the 80 per cent of women who can use them is still in doubt. They change somewhat the quality of the mucus that is normally present in the slitlike cavity of the uterus. This difference in the uterine fluid doubtless deters to some extent progress through it of spermatozoa on their way to the tubes, in one or another of which there may lie an egg in wait for them. There is no doubt that at least on occasion enough succeed in making the trip.

When they do, and conception takes place, the fate of the new human organism is in doubt. We know that it normally takes four days for it to be moved into the uterus. During this time the original single-cell, fertilized egg prepares itself to gain access to the mother's blood vessels that have been especially developed for its benefit in the lining of the womb. From dependable animal studies it seems quite probable that if the young embryo arrives in the uterine cavity too soon, it dies before it has acquired the ability to tap a blood vessel. Also, if it arrives behind time, the outer layer of its cells that had been ready to do this on time have changed in such a way as now to be ineffective; Or the whole organism may have suffered deadly damage by loss of the natural nourishment it was meant to get earlier. In either event, an acceleration or retardation of arrival of the conceptus in the womb would very likely mean harmful, if not fatal, interference with its normal development. There is some experimental evidence to suggest that stimulation, by the inlying IUD, of contractions in the muscular uterine wall, spread to cause change in the function of the muscle fibers in the attached tubes through which the egg passes. It is contractions in these that normally control the passage and the timing of progress of spermatozoa upward from the womb, and of the egg downward into it. A few studies appear to show that the IUD so modifies muscular action as to militate strongly against properly timed meeting and jointure of germ cells. It has, however, also been suggested that the birth control efficacy of the IUD is exercised not really contraceptively but rather by interference with normal implantation of the embryo by disturbing the delicately adjusted timing of its settling on the lining of the womb. Further study will tell. It is an important question, for there are many people in various cultures who view as an abortion any destruction, by any means, of the embryo, however young. Among these groups, the natural human repugnance to abortion would surely deprive the IUD of general acceptability for reduction of population growth.

Unfortunately there are other untoward results that render not wholly acceptable this very effective birth control method, even among those who would not object to an exceedingly early abortion, if this were the only alternative to full pregnancy. In a few, but still too many women, the plastic device causes the lining of the womb on which it rests to bleed troublesomely, or it evokes uncomfortable cramps that arouse apprehension or are unbearably severe. Women so affected feel its removal to be obligatory. From some others it is spontaneously rejected by uterine contractions. These subjects make up most of the 20 per cent for whom the IUD is not useful.

It has certain advantages over the pill. It costs but a fraction of a cent to manufacture. Once the decision has been made to adopt it, no further volition is required for as many months or years as it remains in place. But, like the pill, the IUD also requires medical attention. Its placement is not to be entrusted to either physicians or paramedical persons who are not thoroughly conversant with the proper technique. The uterine cavity is often elusive, and the uterine wall is too easily punctured by anyone who has not had the necessary training. Periodic examination to make sure the device remains in proper place is not always easy for the patient herself to do accurately. In such case she must be examined every now and then by a professional person. It must be said, however, that the amount of medical attention required by the IUD is rather less than the comforting supervision needed for happy use of the pill.

Notwithstanding the frustrating impediments in the way of nationwide utilization of the apparently harmless and exceedingly effective IUD, the United Nations Commission urged the government of India immediately to undertake a vigorous, nationwide crusade in its favor, because of the relief it would give to enormous numbers of parents—very poor and largely illiterate—and so to the country at large. These careful, able, conscientious investigators concluded that this method would be gladly accepted by many millions of women now despairing of relief from family-destructive misery or even famine. If effectively distributed and applied during the next decade, the Commission estimated the growth rate by use of the IUD would be cut by 40 per cent.

It did not advise the Indian government regarding the pill, for unlike the other methods I have discussed, the pill in 1965, when the Commission made its recommendations, had not received the now current government approval for its general use as a contraceptive. Since, when used properly, the pill is 100 per cent effective and fully applicable to the enormous numbers of literate citizens, its widespread use would without doubt diminish the growth rates by, I would judge, at least 40 per cent.

If all three of these big guns—sterilization, the pill, and the IUD—hit the target, and were effectively supported by increase of the marriage age and the condom, the growth of population in

India, after ten years, would approach a standstill. Thereby, plus all the food that developed nations can supply her, India could, in the sad words of the authoritative population experts, "reduce the severity of the oncoming famine during the next decade."

When the growth rate in all developing nations is similarily diminished, endeavors to raise the standard of living—education, transportation, communication, water supply, sewerage, and all that makes possible the welfare of our species—could reach the level merited by the now half-starved and largely illiterate superior human beings, whose true purpose in life is to safeguard the continued evolution of our intellectuality.

Here and there I have spoken about motivation, about medical and paramedical personnel, about illiteracy and ignorance. I have discussed effective methods to break the otherwise automatic connection between copulation and procreation. These are all theoretically acceptable. Properly used they are all individually and socially harmless. Why then does our already excessive global growth rate continue to accelerate faster than food production can possibly increase in time to save from lethal starvation masses of the already distressed inhabitants of South America, India, and of other parts of Southeast Asia? It is because these methods are unknown or unavailable to parents who so desperately need them. They sadly lack motivating knowledge, or as yet these methods are not at their disposal.

Of course continued vigorous research is called for, that better contraceptive methods can be discovered. Of equal importance right now is an all-out effort on the part of developed nations to train enough personnel, from within every half-starving country, to work among their people. But even they could accomplish nothing without facilities, which their countries are too impoverished to supply. This absolute requirement, we of the favored nations must strive to meet. Even among us, both here and abroad, there is lamentable dearth of teaching facilities and of teachers to use them. The over-all job of securing species-welfare is enormous. We, too, need realization and motivation. If the tremendous resources of developed nations are not pitifully wasted on wars to protect each of us from stupid, self-defeating covetousness in ourselves or others, there will be plenty of money for us all to do our part in this war against social destruction. The United Nations is splendidly engaged in the grand effort to make all countries charitably considerate of the welfare of each other. Only thus can any one of us achieve the peaceful strength of our people that will enable us all to approach the universal spiritual goal of humanity—ultimate Truth. On the welfare of each depends the security of all.

NOTE ON CONTRIBUTOR

John Rock (M.D., 1915, Harvard Medical School) is founder and director of the Rock Reproductive Clinic, Brookline, Massachusetts and gynecologist and surgeon at the Parkway Division of the Boston Hospital for Women. He serves as secretary of the Foundation for Reproductive Research and is clinical professor emeritus of gynecology, at Harvard University and honorary surgeon, Massachusetts General Hospital, Boston. His many national and international honors include the Modern Medicine Award for Distinguished Achievement and LL.D. (Hon.) Harvard University. With Dr. Ramon-Garcia and based on collaborative research with the late Gregory Pincus of the Worcester Foundation for Experimental Biology, Dr. Rock was the first to test the effectiveness of oral contraceptives in the now classical studies in Puerto Rico. He is the author of the highly influential book for laymen on birth control, *The Time Has Come.*

4

Antibiotics: Curative Drugs

LOUIS WEINSTEIN, PH.D., M.D.

THE TERM *antibiotic* is derived from the word *antibiosis,* which translated literally means *against life.* This phenomenon has surely operated since there first existed two living forms that competed for survival and perpetuation of the species. One destroyed the other to use it for food; or the weaker of the two perished because it lost out in a struggle for a common source of nourishment or a mutually desirable place in which to live and breed. The term *antibiosis* was first used in 1881 by Viullemin, who described his concept of it in these words:

The lion that springs on its prey and the serpent that poisons the wound before devouring its victim are not considered to be parasites. There is nothing unequivocal about it—one creature destroys the life of another in order to sustain its own, the first being entirely active and the second entirely passive; one is in unrestricted opposition to the other. The relation is so simple that it has never been named, but instead of being examined in isolation it can be viewed as a factor in more complex phenomena. For simplicity we shall refer to it as *antibiosis;* the active participant will be the *antibiote.*

Antibiosis exists throughout the macrocosm and microcosm, the inhabitants of which prey on each other and do not restrict their activities to their own world. The need to survive forces

[70]

viruses to prey on bacteria, plants, and animals. Bacteria attack practically all other living forms to obtain sustenance and to reproduce. Molds or fungi parasitize other species for the same reasons. Higher animals prey on each other and on almost all lower forms to maintain themselves and increase their kind. Even man, the highest level of animal life, in unreasonable moments may become an antibiote for other members of his species. In its broadest definition then, antibiosis exists throughout the biological world. While this phenomenon is obviously impossible *without life,* life itself could not be sustained without antilife. My discussion involves a restricted area of this phenomenon, one that applies only to the activity of some molds and bacteria against other molds and bacteria. That such antagonism is due to chemical compounds elaborated by these organisms was first suggested in 1885 by two French workers, Cornil and Babes. These substances are now known as *antibiotics,* a term coined in 1942 by Selman Waksman, the discoverer of streptomycin. These are the tools for the modern treatment of infection.

The attempt to use substances derived from one organism to inhibit others is almost as old as the science of bacteriology. The medical application of this phenomenon, without appreciation of its nature, is, in fact, very much older. The Chinese were aware over 2,500 years ago of the curative properties of moldy curd of soybeans applied to boils, carbuncles, and similar infections. For a great many years medical literature has contained accounts of the beneficial effects of soil and various plants in certain kinds of localized infections. These were probably due to antibiotics present in these materials. The first suggestion that antagonism between bacteria might be of importance in the treatment of disease was made in 1877 by Pasteur and Joubert. They noticed that the bacteria responsible for an animal and human infection called *anthrax* grew rapidly when placed in sterile urine, but they died if one of the so-called *common air bacteria* was introduced at the same time. When they performed the same experiment in animals, disease did not develop. This was the first clear cut demonstration of an antibiotic effect. It is interesting that these investigators remarked that this phenomenon might hold "great promise for therapeutics." Late in the nineteenth and early in the twentieth century several substances that suppressed the growth of bacteria were discovered, and some were even tested in patients. However, they were too toxic and had to be discarded. Another approach to the treatment of infections utilizing the antagonistic activity of one organism against another was attempted in the 1880's. This was called *replacement therapy* and involved inoculation of non-disease-producing bacteria into patients invaded by disease-producing ones. This method was actually used with some degree of success in the therapy of such diseases as diphtheria, tuberculosis, and plague. All attempts to develop an antibiotic that could cure infections without serious injury to people were unsuccessful until penicillin was discovered.

In 1928 Sir Alexander Fleming, working in the Bacteriology Department of St. Mary's Hospital in London, noticed that a culture of the pus-producing organism, the staphylococcus, was disappearing in the area where a green mold, probably carried on the dust blown in from Praed Street, was growing. This mold belonged to the species *Penicillium*. Its ability to kill bacteria had actually been observed thirty-seven years earlier, in 1881, by another Briton, Tyndall, who in a publication entitled *Essays on the Floating Matter of the Air* described the clearing of solutions clouded by bacterial growth when species of *Penicillium* grew on the surface of the liquid. He failed to go beyond this simple observation. However, Fleming quickly associated the phenomenon that he had observed with what Pasteur and Joubert had earlier referred to as "great promise for therapeutics." He named the substance that he thought responsible for inhibition of bacterial growth *penicillin*. Although Fleming tried to treat human infections, the results were not encouraging because of the low degree of potency and the instability of the material he had. It was not until eleven years later in 1939 that the pressure of war with its huge number of infected wounds stimulated

Florey, Chain, and Abraham at Oxford University to re-examine the possibility that penicillin might be produced in large enough quantity and in a form sufficiently stable to treat human disease. By 1941 they accumulated enough of the antibiotic to begin treatment of serious infections. The results were dramatic, and patients doomed to die made rapid and complete recoveries when given penicillin. However, the drug was so crude and of such weak activity that over one hundred quarts of broth were required to make enough for one patient for one day. Bedpans were actually used to grow the cultures of the antibiotic-producing mold. The first patient reported by the Oxford group was a policeman with a lethal infection. He was given penicillin, some of which had been recovered from the urine of other patients who had received the drug, and survived. Learning this, an Oxford professor is said to have referred to penicillin as a remarkable substance grown in bedpans and purified by passage through the Oxford Police Force.

Commercial manufacture of penicillin on a large scale was impossible in Great Britain because of the exigencies of World War II. However, an extensive research program involving government, university, and industrial laboratories was initiated in the United States. Methods for large-scale production, purification, and stabilization were developed rapidly, and clinical trials were carried out with such dispatch that by the summer of 1943 five hundred cases had been treated with penicillin in this country, and the drug was adopted for use in all of the medical services of the United States Armed Forces. By the end of 1948 large amounts of this antibiotic were being produced. Thus, in about seven years, penicillin developed from an interesting substance made in pitifully small quantities in a university laboratory to a highly effective and truly indispensable therapeutic agent manufactured by drug firms in pure form and in enormous quantities. This marked the beginning of the modern era of the treatment of infection, or what has been called the *golden age of chemotherapy.*

The remarkable effectiveness of penicillin prompted an intensive search for other antibiotics. It was quite natural that this should turn first to the soil, because it had been known for many years that the stability of the microbial population of the soil was, in some way, controlled and maintained by antagonism among the multitude of bacteria and molds it contained. So in 1944 Selma Waksman, a noted soil microbiologist, reported the discovery of the next useful antibiotic. This was made by a species of bacteria called *Streptomyces griseus* and was named *streptomycin*. This drug was effective against a number of bacteria not affected by penicillin; most significantly, it was active against the organism responsible for tuberculosis. The development of this antibiotic was the result of a well-planned, scientifically directed effort and stands in sharp contrast to the pure chance finding of penicillin. Since 1944, a large number of other antibiotics have been developed by using this approach. Most of them are made by bacteria and fungi which have been obtained from soil. Progress in this field has been startling in its breadth and significance for human disease. The discovery and development of the antibiotics has been considered by some to be the most significant medical contribution up to this point in the twentieth century and to be as important as the discovery of anesthesia or the development of the science of bacteriology in the nineteenth century.

The search for new agents of value in the therapy of infections has continued at a high level of activity. Evidence for this is the fact that, of the funds expended in 1965 by twenty-one companies on research and development of all types of drugs, 18.6 per cent or 39 million dollars was spent on anti-infective compounds alone. This was exceeded only by the cost of research for substances to treat diseases of the nervous system and was about equal to the total money spent for discovery of agents that might be effective in hormone disorders, metabolic disturbances, and cancer (Table 1).

TABLE I

*Applied Research and Development Spending
in 1965 by Drug Firms
Surveyed by Pharmaceutical Manufacturers Association*

Human Use	Firms Reporting	Spending (millions)	Per Cent of all Spending
Central Nervous System	37	$37.1	20.4
Parasitic and Infective Diseases	21	33.9	18.6
Neoplasms, Endocrine System, and Metabolic Diseases	27	32.8	18.0
Cardiovascular System	36	18.8	10.3
Other Pharmaceuticals	25	18.5	10.1
Digestive or Genito-urinary Systems	32	15.1	8.3
Biological Products	13	8.4	4.6
Respiratory System	26	5.5	3.0
Vitamins, Nutrients, and Hematinics	17	4.6	2.5
Diagnostic Agents	20	4.0	2.2
Skin	17	3.4	1.9
Total	42	$182.1	100%

From a single antibiotic in 1942, we now have available at least thirty-seven such drugs for human use, and this number will undoubtedly increase over the years. The quantity of these compounds produced in the United States for medical purposes is

staggering. Information furnished by the Chemical Division of
the United States Tariff Commission indicates that 455,000
pounds of penicillin were manufactured in 1955, 859,000 pounds
in 1960 and 1961, 749,000 pounds in 1965. These are astronomical amounts if one considers the relatively small quantity
required to treat most infections. In 1960, 287,000 pounds of
tetracycline compounds were produced; in 1965, this rose to
2,544,750 pounds. The magnitude of this is emphasized by the
fact that a little less than one ounce of one of these drugs is
consumed in two weeks of treatment with a conventional dose.
Since most tetracycline capsules contain 250 mg. or about 0.008
of an ounce of the drug, 2,544,750 pounds represent about five
billion capsules, or about twenty-five for every man, woman, and
child in our population of approximately 200,000,000. The length
of an average tetracycline capsule is about three-fourths of an
inch. On this basis, all of the tetracycline manufactured in 1965,
if placed in capsules and laid end-to-end, would extend for about
60,000 miles, one-fourth of the distance to the moon or about
two and one-half times around the world. The total quantities of
all antibiotics made for human use in 1955 was 79,000,000
pounds; in 1960, 114,000,000 pounds; and in 1965, 162,000,-
000 pounds.

TABLE 2

Quantities of Antibiotics Manufactured
in the United States for Human Use

	POUNDS		
Year	Penicillin	Tetracycline	All Antibiotics
1955	455,000	————	79,000,000
1960	859,000	287,000	114,000,000
1965	1,749,000	2,544,750	162,000,000

Examination of the cost experiences of hospital pharmacies discloses the extent to which antibiotics are used. In a recent survey we found that one hospital spends $7,000 per month or 30 per cent of its total outlay for drugs, just for these compounds. Two other hospital pharmacies reported that 20 and 40 per cent respectively of all their expenditures were for this one group of agents.

TABLE 3

Hospital Expenditures
for Antibiotics

Hospital	Cost of All Drugs	Cost of Antibiotics	% of Total Drug Costs
A	$ 63,000	$21,000	30
B	$ 65,000	$26,000	40
C	$300,000	$60,000	20

The manufacture of such huge quantities of antibiotics reflects the need and demand for them, and attests to their usefulness in the management of most infectious diseases. Unlike these agents, practically all the other drugs in use today do not cure but merely alleviate or eliminate the symptoms of various disorders. So, digitalis improves heart failure but does not alter the disease that produced it. The tranquilizers take the edge off psychoneuroses or make the frankly insane person more manageable, but do not eradicate the responsible basic disturbances. Aspirin makes life bearable for the patient with arthritis, but does not repair his sick joints. Insulin controls diabetes, but does not remove its cause. Despite its reputation as a miracle drug, cortisone does not actually cure a single disorder for which it is employed. The antibiotics are, on the other hand, truly curative. By eliminating the cause, they restore people with infections to a normal state of health which does not require repeated or continuous exposure to

them. There are only a few other drugs that actually cure;
mercury in syphilis, quinine and several other agents in malaria,
and certain compounds in some worm infestations. It is noteworthy that all of these illnesses are infections, and the compounds used to treat them, like the antibiotics, eliminate the
cause of the disease.

The effectiveness of the antibiotics as curative agents is readily
apparent when one compares the death rates of some of the
common infections in the preantibiotic era with those in the
"golden age of chemotherapy." For example, the fatality rate in a
very common kind of pneumonia caused by a bacterium called
the *pneumococcus* was recorded as ranging from 20 to 85 per
cent in the 1941 edition of an authoritative textbook on medicine. It was very high when certain complications developed. The
comment was made that people over seventy years of age rarely
recovered. The 1963 edition of the same book records the risk of
death from this disease, in cases treated with an antibiotic, as only
about 5 per cent. Today a great many people in their seventies
with this kind of pneumonia survive. Practically 100 per cent of
persons who developed an infection of the heart valves called
subacute bacterial endocarditis prior to 1945 died. Proper antibiotic treatment for about one month has now reduced the death
rate in this disease to about 5 per cent. The outlook for uncomplicated recovery in three common forms of meningitis has been
altered most strikingly by treatment with these drugs. One of
these, due to a bacterium called *Hemophilus influenzae* and commonest in young children, was fatal in 100 per cent of cases
before antibiotics were available; treated early with the proper
drugs, less than 5 per cent of these babies now die. The death
rate in meningitis caused by the pneumococcus was 100 per cent
before the advent of penicillin. Over the past twenty years, only
about 8 per cent of a large number of patients with this disease,
whom we have treated, have failed to survive. Epidemic spinal
meningitis, produced by a bacterium called the *meningococcus,*
killed between 20 and 90 per cent of its untreated victims; anti-

biotic therapy has now reduced this to 1 to 2 per cent. The chance of death from typhoid fever, a disease still very common in many of the underdeveloped areas of the world, has been reduced from 8 to 10 to 1 to 2 per cent by the use of an antibiotic, chloramphenicol (Chloromycetin).

TABLE 4

Effects of Antibiotics on
Death Rates of Several
Common Infections

	% Deaths	
Diseases	*No Antibiotics*	*Antibiotic Therapy*
Pneumonia (Pneumococcal)	20-85	About 5
Subacute Bacterial Endocarditis	99+	5
Meningitis H. influenzae	100	2-3
Meningitis (Pneumococcus)	100	8-10
Meningitis Epidemic Spinal (Meningococcal)	20-90	1-5
Typhoid Fever	8-10	1-2

Although the risks of death from certain infections have been remarkably reduced by treatment with antibiotics, the over-all value of these drugs does not rest nor can it be judged on this basis alone. Their effects in decreasing the incidence of complications and duration of illness, and even preventing a great many of the common infectious disorders are even more striking. For example, three infections caused by the streptococcus have been converted from somewhat prolonged, uncomfortable, and potentially dangerous experiences to mild diseases of short duration and benign outcome by treatment with penicillin. Thus "strep sore throat," a disease often featured by high fever and severe discomfort in swallowing, usually persisted for a week or more and was frequently complicated by quinsy, ear infections, and mastoiditis before antibiotics were available. Now penicillin therapy allows uncomplicated recovery in two to three days in practically all instances. Not too many years ago patients with scarlet fever, another common illness due to the streptococcus, were isolated for three to four or more weeks in the hospital, developed a large variety of complications, and when they returned home to their families who had been quarantined for varying periods, often infected their brothers and sisters. The use of penicillin has changed all this. Isolation is now for only forty-eight hours, families are no longer jailed in their homes, and, after two to four days of treatment patients are able to return to work or school, where they are no danger to their associates. Erysipelas, a disease of the skin also due to the streptococcus, occurs most frequently in older people. Untreated it is often severe and may cause death. Penicillin treatment produces rapid recovery and the recurrences that used to develop in about 20 per cent of cases are no longer a problem.

The impact of the antibiotics on the venereal diseases has been tremendous. Before penicillin was available, eradication of syphilis involved one or sometimes two years of weekly injections of an arsenic compound. This long period of treatment discouraged many patients; some dropped out before they were rid of the disease, and not only endangered their survival, but also constituted a public health menace. Persons with involvement of the heart, brain, and spinal cord were difficult to cure and were prone to severe and even fatal drug reactions. So remarkable have been the changes brought about by penicillin in syphilis that the label "miracle drug" would be justified if this were the only disease it cured. One injection a day for ten days of a special preparation of penicillin cures all uncomplicated cases of syphilis. When the brain or spinal cord is affected, the only additional therapy is extension of the period of treatment to fifteen days. Tetracycline is an adequate substitute in patients sensitive to penicillin. The effects of antibiotics in gonorrhea are just as impressive. The severe discomfort of the acute phase of the disease and the distressing and sometimes dangerous manifestations of the chronic stage are effectively controlled and eliminated by penicillin therapy.

Most infections of the lungs, except those caused by true viruses, are cured by antibiotics. Pneumonia due to the pneumococcus heals rapidly when penicillin or other drugs are administered. Other types of pneumonia caused by various bacteria are also well controlled by properly selected antibiotics. Primary atypical pneumonia and psittacosis, a disease contracted from birds and known as *parrot fever,* respond effectively to treatment with one of the tetracyclines. Tuberculosis, still a common disease in the United States and very prevalent in the underdeveloped areas of the world, has undergone a complete metamorphosis since compounds that suppress the growth of or kill the tubercle bacillus have been developed. Streptomycin was the first drug to produce a significant impact on this disease. Although this agent is still employed as adjunct therapy in severe tuberculosis, the drugs presently used most widely are not antibiotics.

Boils and more life-threatening infections due to the pus-forming bacterium, the staphylococcus, respond remarkably well when an adequate dose of an effective antibiotic is administered. About fifteen years ago the staphylococcus began to develop resistance to penicillin and other antibiotics. Infections due to this organism became increasingly difficult to treat successfully, and the death rate from severe disease of this kind began to approach that experienced in the preantibiotic era. Fortunately, several agents active against these resistant staphylococci have recently become available and have rapidly and effectively reversed this trend. Some of these drugs are new forms of penicillin; others are chemically different compounds. The acute stage of infections of the kidneys and bladder is readily suppressed by moderate doses of one of several drugs given for ten to twelve days. Chronic disease of this type is difficult to cure but can be controlled by treatment over an extended period. Many other infections can be cured by antibiotics.

In addition to their effectiveness in curing established infections and saving life, the antibiotics are also of great value in preventing some infectious diseases. For example, a patient with a "strep throat" or scarlet fever need not endanger the other members of his family, because if they are given modest doses of penicillin or erythromycin by mouth for five days, they will remain well. Knowledge of a venereal contact, which may have exposed an individual to gonorrhea, allows the physician to prevent this disease by the early administration of penicillin or a tetracycline compound. Giving an antibiotic to which the bacterium that causes dystentery is sensitive to healthy contacts may bring a developing epidemic of this infection to an abrupt halt. When persons with heart damage who require dental or other types of surgery are given penicillin for a short period before and after operation, they may avoid the heart valve infection, subacute bacterial endocarditis. Antibiotics are also of prophylactic value in people with some noninfectious diseases that may recur or be complicated by infection. The individual whose heart has been injured by rheumatic fever may be spared further attacks of this disease, with added harm to this organ, by taking penicillin daily for a long period or, as has been suggested by some, for the rest of his life. The prolonged survival of children with a disease known as cystic fibrosis of the pancreas is, in no small part, attributable to the daily administration of an antibiotic. This decreases markedly their tendency to get pneumonia, a complication that, in the preantibiotic era, usually snuffed out their life at a very young age.

A critical evaluation of the total impact of antibiotics requires more than mere consideration of their activity on infection itself, for this omits examination of the roles they play in improving other aspects of illness. Such disease often involves serious and distressing socioeconomic upheaval for patients, and important public health problems for their families and friends. Many persons with readily curable infections can now be treated at home and are spared the extended periods of hospitalization required not so long ago. The financial savings in terms of the present costs of hospital care for the millions of people who suffer this kind of disease in the United States each year must be huge. In addition, rapid cure allows people to return to work much earlier than before, and so they are not afflicted with the burden of lack of income because of prolonged illness. Taken together, the economic impact of these "ripple" effects of antibiotic therapy, although not accurately calculable, are undoubtedly tremendous. Other benefits of antibiotic treatment include (a) reduction of the social disruption that may result from the removal of one of the parents, especially the mother, from the home to the hospital and (b) avoidance of the psychological trauma incident to hospitalization, especially in young children.

The public health benefits of antibiotic therapy are striking when its accomplishments in the control of some of the so-called communicable diseases are examined. Treatment of "strep sore throat" with penicillin, by eradicating the responsible bacteria from the patient, decreases the risk of his spreading this infection to others and prevents the development of epidemics. There are, in many communities, a variable number of people harboring the bacterium responsible for diphtheria. These so-called carriers are the sources from which nonimmune individuals contract this disease. Until antibiotics became available, little could be done to alter this dangerous situation. Now, about two weeks of treatment with penicillin or erythromycin eliminates the carrier state. A similar situation exists with respect to *Salmonella,* organisms that cause food poisoning. Healthy carriers of these bacteria are often responsible for large outbreaks of this disease because they contaminate food that they prepare or handle. Until a short time ago no drug capable of eradicating these organisms from all such individuals was available. However, a recently developed antibiotic called *ampicillin* now accomplishes this in many cases. By reducing the number of Salmonella carriers its use may decrease the risk of epidemics of food poisoning.

In no situation is the effect of antibiotics in preventing disease, reducing suffering, saving life, and returning the victims of infection to activity more dramatic than in war. A review of the medical experiences of the War between the States, the Spanish-American War, and World Wars I and II indicates that (a) infections killed more soldiers than bullets in some of these campaigns and (b) infected wounds accounted for a great many deaths and much of the incapacitation from duty. Comparison of the later stages of the second World War, the Korean episode, and the present conflict in Vietnam with these earlier wars brings out the tremendous improvement in the impact and outcome of infections that has been brought about by the antibiotics. It has been stated that in no other military encounter has the salvage rate from wounds approached that presently being observed in Southeast Asia. Although rapid removal of the wounded from the battlefield to hospitals and highly skilled surgical treatment are mainly responsible for this, antibiotics, by preventing and curing infections that complicate such dreadful injuries, undoubtedly contribute considerably to this excellent experience.

One of the very important accomplishments of modern medicine has been a significant increase in life expectancy. This is mostly due to a sharp decrease in the death rate among young children. Improved nutrition, repair of correctable birth defects, treatment of chemical disturbances, and routine immunization have played a crucial role in the young. However, antibiotic therapy of infections, very common events in this age group, has also saved the lives of countless youngsters and allowed them to grow to adulthood. Only a small increment has been added to the length of survival of older people. There has been no significant improvement in their chances for survival from cancer, strokes, and heart attacks. The small increase in life expectancy that the elderly are experiencing is due, in considerable degree, to our ability to cure infections to which they are prone, and which in the past carried them off with dispatch and in great numbers.

This long recital of the benefits of antibiotic therapy prompts inquiry into the mechanisms by which cure of infection is accomplished. Two factors operate to bring about this result: (a) Injury to bacteria by the drugs and (b) the anti-infection defenses of the patient. Antibiotics interfere with some of the essential life processes of bacteria. Some, like penicillin, make it impossible for them to form a cell wall, a relatively rigid structure that protects them against inimical factors in their external environment. Others, the tetracyclines for example, interfere in one way or another with the ability of organisms to make protein, a defect that causes them to stop multiplying or to die. Despite their direct antibacterial activities, antibiotics may fail to eradicate infections. This occurs most often in persons who are unable to mobilize or who are deficient in certain inherent defense mechanisms. Such people cannot contribute the essential factors necessary for final cure of infection, and as a result, respond very slowly to treatment or die.

The antibiotic coin is not all glitter. It also has its dark side. All of these drugs have the capacity for harm. The frequency and severity of the reactions they produce varies with each compound, and to some degree, with the person treated. All antibiotics produce allergic responses. Some of these are mild, but others are very severe and may even be fatal; for example, death has followed a single injection of penicillin in persons sensitized to this substance. Various kinds of skin rashes may develop during use of any of these agents. Some antibiotics are inherently toxic and damage the ears, kidneys, liver, and the blood. A few cause nausea, vomiting, and diarrhea when taken by mouth. All, when given in conventional doses, alter the numbers and types of bacteria normally present in the nose, throat, and lower intestinal tract. Most people suffer no ill effects from such changes; a few are infected by their own bacteria. In this instance the drug, while curing one infection, provokes the development of another, which may be more severe and life-threatening than the one for which treatment was given initially. The list of reactions produced by antibiotics is long and dreary in the amount of disease and suffering induced. When untoward effects appear in situations in which antibiotic therapy is mandatory, they are acceptable as the price for cure. However, when they follow unnecessary use of these drugs, they are totally unacceptable.

The tendency for some bacteria to lose their susceptibility to antibiotics presents an increasingly frequent and difficult problem. Among the drug resistant species are the staphylococcus, Salmonella, and the dysentery bacillus. Even the bacterium that causes gonorrhea is now less sensitive to penicillin than it was twenty years ago. The existence of such organisms has created many difficulties in the therapy of the diseases they cause. In some cases the development of new antibiotics has solved the problem, at least temporarily. In a number of others no such solution is presently available.

The glamour of the antibiotics, as emphasized not only in the medical literature but to an unusual degree in the lay press, has been responsible for a number of misconceptions about their capabilities. The present state of information concerning these compounds is a mixture of fact and fancy not only in the minds of the laity, but even in those of some physicians. Up to this point I have been discussing what we believe to be fact. Now I would like to comment on a few of what I consider to be fancies concerning these drugs.

The notion that antibiotics will prevent or cure all infections and that no one need acquire or die of this kind of disease is wrong. Also erroneous is the impression that these drugs are of value in treating and preventing the complications of the common cold and other virus infections of the respiratory tract. No significant advantage accrues from the use of two, three, or four antibiotics at the same time, in most instances. While a few infections fare best when two or rarely three of these drugs are given simultaneously, in most cases the best results are accomplished with the least danger when an adequate dose of a single effective antibiotic is administered. The practice of treating with antibiotics such common childhood diseases as chicken pox, mumps, and measles when they are uncomplicated is the height of fancy, for there is absolutely no evidence that they are benefited in any way by these drugs. The idea that no more than a single dose or one or two days of use of one of these drugs is needed to cure mild infections is not supported by experience. This practice often leads to a sequence of relapses and remissions that is interrupted only when treatment is finally carried out for a sufficiently long time. With few exceptions the minimal period of therapy required is one week; in some diseases this must be extended to two or four or more weeks. The administration of an antibiotic to try to control fever for which no cause is apparent represents one of the greatest and most frequent misuses of these agents. Most short-lived fevers are due to virus infections, for which these compounds are valueless. Even when a significant fever has persisted for several weeks, antibiotics should not be given empirically. The presence of a troublesome degree of fever demands careful medical study to elicit its cause and not a barrage of drugs given in the hope, usually futile, that one of them will accomplish a return of the temperature to normal.

The medical profession is often accused of indiscriminate use of antibiotics. While this may be true in some cases, not a small part of this problem is the direct fault of patients themselves. Many people are so convinced of the omnipotence of these drugs that they insist on their administration. If their physician, in his good judgment, refuses their demand, they threaten him with seeking out another doctor, who under unrelenting pressure, may satisfy their compulsion for treatment. In the same class are the persons who have a stock of antibiotics in their medicine cabinets. These are usually "left-over" compounds, which have been effective when prescribed by a physician at some prior time. At the first sign of illness that suggests the possibility of infection, usually fever, one or more of the stocked drugs is taken by a parent, or given by him to his child. This is an extremely dangerous practice. Antibiotics must never be taken without medical direction. Self-medication of this type is much more likely to produce harm than good and must be severely condemned.

An erroneous concept common among some physicians is that a newly developed antibiotic represents progress. This is sometimes not true, because the new drug may not be as good as the claims that are made for it. Wide substitution of such an unproved agent for others of documented value and safety may actually represent a backward step in the treatment of infection. Considerable time is required before any antibiotic can be accurately evaluated. The development of our knowledge of the usefulness of every one of these drugs usually progresses through three well-defined stages. The first might be called the *Stage of Hyperenthusiasm*. This encompasses the first two or three years after a drug becomes available. During this period the medical literature is devoted to a catalogue of all of the benefits associated with its use, with only an occasional reference to reactions or failure of response. The next three to five years cover a period that might be labeled the *Stage of Critical Evaluation*. During this, sufficiently large numbers and varieties of infections are treated, careful clinical and bacteriological studies are carried out, and the results are critically analyzed. During these two stages a large enough experience is usually accumulated to permit determination of the degree of effectiveness and the types and frequency of reactions that may be associated with the use of the drug. Only after five or six or more years of study of an antibiotic is enough learned about it to allow it to be applied most effectively and with the least danger. At this time it might be considered to have reached the *Stage of Known Value*.

The development of the antibiotics has solved a great many problems. However, as is often the case, new problems have rapidly replaced the old ones. This is a very small price to pay for a group of substances, which with very few exceptions are the only truly curative drugs available to the physician. Despite the large number of antibiotics presently at hand, more are required (a) to combat viral infections for which we now have no effective agents, (b) to solve the increasing difficulties associated with the development of bacterial drug resistance and (c) to combat the diseases caused by molds and fungi for the therapy of which there is at this time only one effective compound.

Antibiotics must always be used with circumspection and discrimination. They should be administered only in situations in which they are known to be useful and avoided in those in which indication for their application is entirely lacking, or at best only suggestive. To do otherwise is to expose patients to the risk of reactions that may be more deadly than the infections from which they suffer. These drugs are not universally applicable, nor are they entirely beneficial, and most significant from the standpoint of those who receive them, they are not completely harmless. There is nevertheless no doubt that the antibiotics deserve the label *miracle drugs*. Their activity in the prevention and cure of a great many infections and in saving life is dramatic. The impact of their use on the socioeconomic distresses and the public health aspects of these diseases has been immeasurably great. That the antibiotics have contributed greatly to a better life for all of us is very clear. That they are the most important medical discovery up to this point in the twentieth century is no exaggeration.

NOTE ON CONTRIBUTOR

Louis Weinstein (Ph.D. in Microbiology, Yale University, 1931, M.D. Boston University, 1943) is associate physician-in-chief and chief of the infectious disease service, New England Medical Center Hospitals, professor of medicine at Tufts University School of Medicine and lectures on infectious disease in the Harvard Medical School. He was first a research fellow and then instructor in bacteriology and immunology, Yale University School of Medicine, 1931–1937. From 1939–1945 he was a research fellow in bacteriology and immunology and instructor to associate professor of medicine from 1945 to 1957 at the Boston University School of Medicine. He was chief of the infectious disease service of the Mass. Memorial Hospitals (Boston, Mass.) from 1947 to 1957. An author of numerous articles and several monographs dealing with the background, recognition, and treatment of infections, he has written chapters on the diagnosis and treatment of infections in the leading textbooks of internal medicine and contributed the comprehensive and authoritative sections on antibiotics and sulfonamides to the world's foremost textbook of pharmacology, Goodman and Gilman's *The Pharmacological Basis of Therapeutics.*

5

The Effects of Drugs on the Unborn Child

SYDNEY S. GELLIS, M.D.

FOR CENTURIES THE unborn child, rolling and twisting about in his inland sea inside his mother, has been considered to be quite safely contained within his environment, protected from the cruel outside world by the waters surrounding him and assured of proper nourishment by his direct pipeline to the placenta. It was thought that the placenta served as a very effective barrier to poisonous substances which could go from the mother to the infant. The ineffectiveness of most agents taken by countless generations of women determined to rid themselves of their unwanted tenants strengthened this belief. Although such poisons did not appear to affect him, numerous beliefs have existed since prehistoric times that evil influences could reach and affect the fetus. These were primarily in the realm of black magic and superstitions, which persist to this day in many parts of the world, including our own. Women continue to believe that the witnessing of deformities during pregnancy can permanently mark the unborn child. There is no scientific basis for such a belief; however, one is no longer certain that the unborn infant is completely isolated from the emotional state of the mother. That these beliefs and superstitions cannot be totally disregarded may be indicated by the recent awareness that the heavy smoker who becomes pregnant has a markedly increased chance of giving birth to an infant who weighs appreciably less than his friend born of a nonsmoking mother, and may be born prematurely instead of at term. Just why this is the case is yet to be determined: Is this due to a direct stunting effect of nicotine upon the growing fetus or is it conceivable that smoking has not been responsible for the growth failure, but that other factors, which of themselves drive a woman to indulge in heavy smoking, may play the primary role? What I am trying to say is that we now know that the placenta is not the perfect control mechanism we once believed it to be, and that perhaps the tense, hyperexcitable, fearful woman or her opposite, the depressed, moody, unhappy woman transmits through the placenta substances with which we are familiar, such as adrenalin or glucose, in excess or in insufficient amounts, which have their own effect on the fetus. It has been accepted that the mother-child relationship during the first few months of the infant's life is critical for the normal future emotional development of the infant. Now we must consider the possibility that the *mother-fetal* emotional relationship may be even more critical and that we must somehow convey the importance of regarding happiness as a gay pregnancy.

Having indicated that the placenta may not be the ideal control mechanism, one that passes those substances benefiting the fetus and holds back those substances that may be harmful, let us move on to specific examples of its defects. I shall limit the discussion to toxic agents or drugs, which by the intestinal route, the lung, or by needle enter the bloodstream of the mother and make their way to the placenta, there to be repelled or granted admission to the circulation of the infant. Interest in toxic agents skyrocketed in 1961 with the first reports of the thalidomide disaster recorded almost at the same time by McBride from Australia and Lenz from Germany. This drug, considered an ideal sedative or hypnotic, valuable primarily for inducing a good night's sleep, was available throughout Europe and seemed especially worthwhile because of its low incidence of undesirable side effects. By great good fortune and the stubbornness of Dr. Frances O. Kelsey of the Food and Drug Administration, who felt that experimental studies of the drug were inadequate, thalidomide had not yet been approved for public use in the United States. A review of the European studies and the properties of this drug could have led to no suspicion of its dangerous effects on the fetus but the appearance in almost epidemic form of deformed newborn infants led to the awareness of the role played by thalidomide. The hallmark of its damage to the fetus is "phocomelia," which means flipperlike extremity, a description of the malformed shortened arms of these babies with hands close to the shoulder, the intervening bone and muscle having become markedly foreshortened. Other abnormalities may be present, such as congenital defects of the heart, the gastrointestinal tract, the kidneys, the ears and hearing. Extremities may be so severely involved that they are almost entirely absent. Thalidomide produced such damage to the fetus if the drug was taken in the first third, or trimester, of pregnancy; after that critical period it had no effect. Figures for the exact incidence of deformed babies resulting from this agent are not available, but estimate between 7,500 and 10,000 are given for Europe alone. Of forty women who had received thalidomide in the first trimester, McBride in careful studies showed that 35 per cent of the infants were abnormal. The incidence of malformations was almost 100 per cent if the drug was taken between the 34th and 45th day after the last menstruation, even when very small amounts were taken over short periods of time. A few cases were reported in the United States in women who had taken the drug while traveling in Europe or who had been given thalidomide by friends returning from abroad.

Thalidomide is thus the most infamous of the teratogenic agents—a word derived from *teratology,* the study of malformations. Teratology is a relatively new science, which has received tremendous impetus during the past few years, primarily because we are not only a medicated society but an overmedicated one. Teratogenic agents produce their harmful effect during the early weeks of pregnancy when organ systems are in the process of formation. Once the system is fully developed, exposure to such agents cannot produce an abnormality. Thus the great danger from drugs occurs during this critical period of organ development. Kelsey points out that, in animal experiments, drug-induced malformations do not occur when the fetus is very young and in its predifferentiation period—that is, before the various organs begin to form. The state of early differentiation is the period of highest risk. As the organs and systems become more highly differentiated they become less capable of being damaged.

Prior to the thalidomide disaster, drugs administered to humans were tested quite extensively, but primarily in the individuals for whom they were intended. Young animals of various species were included in such studies, but little emphasis was given to studies of possible ill effect on the fetus. Since the thalidomide experience, careful studies of all new drugs together with old, well-established drugs have been carried out in a number of species during pregnancy on the very fair assumption that any available drug might easily be taken by women unaware of the fact that they are pregnant. Even after the dangers of thalidomide were known, it took considerable experimentation with pregnant animals to reproduce the phenomena occurring in the human. Administration of the drug to rabbits, rats, and mice indicated that the period of danger in such species was very brief, and that failure to test at the exactly proper point in early pregnancy could result in no obvious deformities.

Numerous other drugs have been viewed with suspicion as potential causes of congenital abnormalities. Approximately 2 per cent of all living newborn infants have abnormalities recognizable at birth, and this percentage increases as infants grow older so that by a year an additional 1 to 2 per cent are shown to have abnormalities that existed at birth but could not be detected.

Genetic or inherited factors may be responsible for some, X-rays for some, and infections for others. German measles during the first trimester of pregnancy, for example, is an important cause. Drugs play their role, but how *frequently* they are responsible is still uncertain. In approximately 90 per cent of the infants born with abnormalities there is today no definite explanation for the defects. The incidence of abnormalities in stillborn babies is much higher than in live-born, ranging in some studies to a high of 20 per cent. Possibly the incidence in spontaneous abortions is even higher, but there are relatively few data available on such fetuses. Although knowledge is increasing in the field of drug-induced abnormalities, and drugs that are important agents in teratology are receiving great attention, little or nothing is known of the possible potentiation of the danger of an apparently harmless drug when it is given in combination with another. Recent surveys have shown that 92 per cent of women studied received one or more drugs during their pregnancy.

Probably the first drug to be definitely associated with the production of abnormalities in the fetus was aminopterin, an anticancer drug, which is a folic acid antagonist and was reported by Thiersch in 1952. Such drugs act by suppressing metabolism and proliferation of cells and thus may produce abnormality in the fetus. In other anticancer agents, such as bisulfan and chlorambucil, results have not been as convincing in the human as in experimental animals. However, the indications for the use of such drugs in the mother are usually quite clear and necessary for maintenance of life. A number of investigators have recommended that when these drugs must be used in a pregnant woman, abortion be carried out.

The list of drugs that may be administered to a pregnant woman and be of potential risk to her unborn child is a long one and cannot be reviewed in detail here. However, the actions of several of these in the production of abnormalities of the fetus or in giving rise to changes which, though not life threatening or very deforming, are worthy of discussion.

First of these are several of the hormonal agents and drugs

used to treat disorders of endocrine glands. The worst offenders have been synthetic progestational agents given during pregnancy for either women who habitually spontaneously abort, or for a woman in whom spontaneous abortion may be occurring. In such instances female infants have been born with external genitalia resembling those of a male infant, apparently due to the fact that during the metabolism of synthetic progestins they may act as testosterone, or male hormone. If the drug is given before the twelfth week of pregnancy, fusion of the labia occurs. If the drug is administered after twelve weeks, enlargement of the clitoris is noted. Of interest is the fact that the natural product progesterone, which can be given intramuscularly only, does not appear to cause masculinization of the fetus and is therefore the drug of choice if treatment is indicated. Female infants who have been masculinized as a result of therapy may require fairly extensive plastic surgery to correct the changes induced by the oral agents.

Cortisone has been viewed with great suspicion as a potential teratogenic agent since it became clear early in the study of this drug that it can regularly produce cleft palate in the fetuses of rats and rabbits to whom it is administered. Although it seems very rarely associated with the formation of cleft palate in the human, it is obvious that it should be avoided if at all possible during the early weeks of pregnancy.

DRUGS FOR TREATMENT OF THYROID DISORDERS IN THE MOTHER

Drugs given to control hyperthyroidism in the pregnant woman may, after the first trimester of pregnancy, interfere with the developing thyroid function of the fetus. Drugs such as iodides, radioactive iodine, perchlorates, thiouracils, and others, passing through the placenta quite freely, inhibit thyroxin production in the thyroid gland of the fetus, thus causing stimulation and increase in the thyroid-stimulating hormone of the pituitary gland. This in turn stimulates an increase in the size of the thyroid, a goiter, which may become so large that it causes the head of the fetus to extend back, thus interfering with its birth or so compressing the trachea and larynx by its enlargement that the infant has difficulty with breathing after birth. In addition, the interference with hormone production of the gland may give rise to the signs and symptoms of underfunctioning or overfunctioning of the thyroid in the infant. Thus any of the agents employed in treatment of goiter or hyperthyroidism in the pregnant woman must be used with great caution, and emphasis should be placed on the administration of the smallest amounts compatible with the mother's state of health. Since radioactive iodine, which is frequently used in studies of the thyroid gland in adults, may produce permanent damage to the gland of the fetus, such tests must be avoided during pregnancy.

NARCOTICS

One of the strangest clinical pictures to be encountered in the newborn infant is that seen in the baby born of a narcotic addict. Although narcotics have not as yet been shown to produce abnormalities in the fetus, they may be life-threatening to the infant after birth. The infant, accustomed inside the mother to the regular passage of morphine or heroin from her bloodstream to his, begins to suffer following his birth from narcotic withdrawal symptoms, similar to those of the addict who has been cut off from his supply of drug. In about twenty-four hours the baby becomes extremely agitated, yawns frequently, perspires profusely, and is very hyperactive, actually crawling about the crib as though in pain. His pupils may be pinpoint in size. His skin becomes flushed, his cry high pitched, shrill, and annoying. He may develop tremors, convulsions, and die, unless the condition is promptly recognized. Treatment may be comparable to that of the adult with narcotic withdrawal symptoms, namely, the administration of decreasing doses of the drug until the infant can be weaned from his dependency on it. Since few women voluntarily reveal their addiction, recognition of the symptoms in the infant is dependent on the physician's familiarity with the condition or suspicion of the mother because of the presence of unexplained needle marks in her skin. Similar clinical findings have been reported in women who have had prolonged treatment with tincture of opium or codeine or women who are alcoholics.

ANTIMICROBIAL AGENTS

Numerous antibiotics and other antimicrobial agents have produced harm to the fetus. Two examples can be cited as illustrations. The first is the popular antibiotic, the tetracyclines, which when administered to the pregnant woman late in pregnancy, may have two undesirable effects on the fetus. The drugs are deposited in pigmented form in the growing bones of the fetus, where they may temporarily produce delayed growth. Even more important, they are deposited in the developing teeth, where they cause discoloration and abnormalities of the enamel. These are not visible until the teeth erupt, when the abnormalities and discoloration are clearly evident. The color, at first yellow, gradually on exposure to light becomes a muddy brown. It is readily differentiated from other causes of dental discoloration by the fact that under exposure to ultraviolent light the teeth fluoresce brightly. The fluorescent change gradually lessens with the passage of time. Although there has been no indication that the administration of tetracyclines to the pregnant woman will produce damage and staining of the permanent teeth, continued administration of these drugs to the infant after birth will produce similar changes in the permanent teeth.

Of much greater significance and risk to the newborn infant is the administration of sulfonamide drugs to the pregnant woman. This is especially true of the long-acting sulfonamides currently in great favor in the treatment of urinary tract infections. The administration of such drugs late in pregnancy may considerably increase the risk of the development in the newborn infant of the condition known as kernicterus. This name is derived from *icterus* meaning jaundice and *kern* meaning kernel or nucleus of the brain. In the past kernicterus has been considered a potential hazard for infants with problems centering around the Rh factor. This form of brain damage is due to bilirubin, the yellow pigment of the blood noted in jaundiced individuals. Bilirubin is released in the destruction of red blood cells, which are constantly breaking down. It passes through the blood stream attached to a protein, albumin, which is always present in the blood serum. When the bilirubin-albumin combination reaches the liver, the bilirubin is detached and excreted in the bile. Bilirubin in the blood stream, which is not attached to albumin, moves out into the tissues. In the brain it acts as a very toxic substance producing damage. Drugs such as the sulfonamides increase the risk of such damage because they attach to albumin more successfully than does bilirubin, leaving the yellow pigment free to move into the brain. The infant who is developing kernicterus or brain damage from bilirubin appears jaundiced. On about the third day of life his sucking reflex begins to deteriorate and he feeds poorly. Next he develops episodes of arching of his neck and back and severe respiratory trouble. Bloody froth appears from nostrils and mouth and death occurs. If the infant survives kernicterus he usually presents the picture of cerebral palsy. Deafness is a frequent result of kernicterus. Thus kernicterus becomes one of the hazards of sulfonamide therapy in pregnancy, especially if the fetus is prematurely born. In the premature infant, levels of albumin are lower than those in full-term infants, and kernicterus occurs even more easily.

Perhaps the most controversial drug at the present time is LSD, for little information is available about its potential hazard to the unborn child. Preliminary studies in pregnant animals suggest that it can produce abnormalities in offspring, and breaks in chromosomes have been noted both in pregnant women on the drug and in their newborn infants. An infant with skeletal deformities has been born of a woman who took LSD at the time during her pregnancy when fetal extremities were beginning development and it is quite possible that LSD was responsible. If additional infants with such abnormalities are born under similar circumstances, the relationship will become quite certain.

Although X-rays cannot be included among the list of drugs that are hazardous to the fetus, we have briefly mentioned previously the necessity for the avoidance of diagnostic or therapeutic procedures during pregnancy employing radioactive iodine, and a brief statement about diagnostic X-rays for the pregnant woman would not seem out of place in this talk. It has long been known that exposure of the pregnant animal or human to X-rays can produce death of the fetus, or if the fetus survives, a number of major abnormalities such as cataracts, tumors, leukemia, or abnormalities of extremities and brain. Again the most devastating of the abnormalities occurs when exposure to X-ray comes during the developmental period of major organs in the embryo. The greatest danger to the fetus results from X-rays taken of the area in which he lies. Thus films of abdomen or pelvis are most likely to affect him. However, X-rays of other portions of the body may still involve the fetus if he has inadequate shielding by lead plates. The more prolonged the X-ray procedure, the greater the hazard. Manipulative procedures under the fluoroscope result in considerably greater exposure than simple X-ray pictures. The older the X-ray equipment, the poorer the shielding devices to protect against stray rays. Clearly it is essential that only such X-ray studies as are absolutely essential should be conducted during pregnancy. Also, since women may have no knowledge that they are pregnant in the very early days following conception, it is an excellent rule to carry out elective X-ray studies in any woman of childbearing age only in the first two weeks following the start of a normal menstruation, thus reducing the risk of unnecessary exposure of the very young embryo.

Up to this point we have mentioned a number of drugs that are relatively uncommon to the experience of the average individual.

You may well ask what is known of the commoner drugs more likely to be found in the bulging medicine cabinet of the citizen of these United States. Barbiturates have been shown to cause excessive bleeding in newborn infants. They of course can, when taken prior to delivery, produce excessive drowsiness and respiratory difficulty in the infant immediately after birth. Several of the antihistamines, remedies against nausea, and antidepressants have been suspected of producing abnormalities. Although the evidence for their teratologic effect is not fully established, sufficient possibility exists to make it unwise for the pregnant woman to receive these agents. Aspirin and other salicylates taken in large amounts have not been shown to produce abnormalities but can produce excessive bleeding in the infant and may, as in the case of the sulfa drugs, increase the risk of brain damage due to kernicterus. Phenacetin which is present in a number of preparations for reduction of fever and achiness may induce excessive breakdown of red blood cells in the fetus or live-born infant. It is also apparent that care must be taken about vitamin preparations, which most of the public tends to forget fall in the field of medications. In a number of instances there appears to be a possible relationship between *excessive* intake of Vitamin D by the pregnant woman and the condition known as hypercalcemia in the young infant. Many laymen believe that if a small amount of a vitamin preparation is a benefit, a great deal will prove even more helpful. In infants with hypercalcemia, as a result of high Vitamin D levels, blood calcium levels are high and abnormalities of the aorta and other major blood vessels of the body are present. These infants have a very fragile, elfin facial appearance, mental retardation, pallor, and vomiting and failure of growth. Exactly the same clinical picture may develop in the young infant who is given excessive doses of Vitamin D. In severely involved infants death ensues as a result of damage to the kidneys. Less severely involved infants may survive but exhibit permanent damage to brain, blood vessels, and skeletal system. All too often, in both pregnant women and young infants, intake of

Vitamin D is excessive. In children and adults who are on well-balanced diets, addition of Vitamin D is entirely unnecessary. Overadministration and self-medication with vitamin preparations by our essentially well-nourished society represent perhaps the most common incidents of overmedication in America today. Owing to the fact that the public does not view these preparations as medications, pregnant women tend to overdose with them and forget to inquire of physicians about the necessity for their ingestion.

There is suspicion but as yet no proof that excessive Vitamin C during pregnancy may result in infants who, despite normal intake of Vitamin C, may develop scurvy; their enzyme systems having adjusted to the need for high levels. A similar case has been argued regarding Vitamin B6, found in many multivitamin preparations, with resulting infants who exhibit repeated, prolonged convulsions unless given daily doses of the vitamin in excess of that found in the normal diet or needed by the normal infant.

Large doses of Vitamin K given prior to the birth of the infant may produce severe anemia with striking increase in incidence of kernicterus because of the hemolyzing or destructive effect of increased levels on the red blood cells of the young infant in the first few days of life with the release of abnormal amounts of the yellow pigment bilirubin.

We have reviewed briefly the role of a number of drugs as teratogenic agents and as causes of abnormal findings in the otherwise normal newborn infant. The medical profession has learned a great deal about these problems in just the past few years, but the information has been slow to reach the public. There must be general awareness of the potential dangers of drugs and especially of the need to end self-medication, which in this country as well as in other parts of the world is on a vast scale. During pregnancy, more than at any other time in the life of a woman, it is vital that no drugs or medication except those specifically prescribed by a physician cognizant of the pregnancy be taken by the patient. Except in life-threatening or disabling situations only those drugs should be given that through long experience have not been found to be involved in the production of abnormalities. No new drug should ever be given to pregnant women unless it represents a great advance in the treatment of important and disabling disorders, and only after it has been thoroughly tested in a variety of pregnant animals. Even under such conditions its use in pregnancy must be carefully controlled and studied, for while some agents may be extremely teratogenic in experimental animals but quite safe for the pregnant female, it is possible that other agents, which prove teratogenic in man, may be harmless in animals. Much more investigational work must be done in the study of simultaneous administration of two or more drugs, because it is not impossible that one may potentiate the toxicity of the other. Although much has been done in studies of the effects of drugs both early and late in pregnancy, more work is needed to determine if there are ill effects during the second trimester or midpregnancy.

In our opening paragraph we mentioned briefly the inland sea in which the unborn child is nourished and protected from the outside world. It is obvious that relatively little is yet known of this sea, and that science has much to do to chart its depths, its shoals and turbulences. As physicians we must do all within our power to maintain its waters calm, untroubled, and safe for its small voyager.

NOTE ON CONTRIBUTOR

Sydney S. Gellis (M.D., 1938, Harvard Medical School) is pediatrician-in-chief at the New England Medical Center Hospitals and professor and chairman of the Department of Pediatrics at Tufts University School of Medicine, Boston, Massachusetts. He holds faculty appointments at all three of Boston's medical schools—Harvard, Boston University, and Tufts. He was a member of the Army Epidemiological Board and consultant to the Secretary of War on infectious diseases during World War II. He serves on the editorial board of the *American Journal of Diseases of Children* and is a member of the special legislative commission on mental retardation for the Commonwealth of Massachusetts.

6

The Drug Approach to Mental Illness

JONATHAN O. COLE, M.D.

Sigmund Freud was probably the first person to work in psychopharmacology in a serious manner, when he involved himself in a study of cocaine. Relatively early in his career he announced in a scientific paper that cocaine was an effective treatment for heroin addiction and that heroin addicts actually liked the drug. A colleague of mine has suggested that one reason Dr. Freud's thoughts and theories about psychoanalysis were so poorly received was not because they were inherently unbelievable, but because he had gone on record with the preposterous claim that cocaine was good for heroin addicts; and anybody who would make that observation on the basis of a small number of cases obviously was fallible and therefore should not be believed. As a matter of fact, Dr. Freud was quite correct in finding that cocaine did have a powerful effect upon mood.

The problem of finding a good drug to treat an organic illness can have several bases; this is true in psychiatric illness as well. Ideally, you should have a drug which prevents an illness or corrects its cause. This is easier said than done in psychiatry, where the causes of most illnesses are currently unknown, and there is no known biological defect to be corrected. Diseases like schizophrenia, depression, even neuroses or chronic alcoholism are believed by some to develop from influences in the environment, from heredity, or from biological abnormalities. The current thought is that these illnesses are produced by some admixture of a variety of social, cultural, environmental, and biological components. In anticipation of finding a more accurate cause of mental illness, one famous Nobel laureate, Dr. Linus Pauling, coined a wonderful phrase, "For every twisted mind, a twisted molecule." Though he may ultimately turn out to be correct, to date the twisted-molecule cause has not been found for most conditions. In fact even if this rather optimistic concept were found to be true, there is certainly no assurance that one could immediately find a drug that would untwist the molecule.

There are, however, some psychiatric illnesses for which there is an etiological treatment—penicillin kills the spirochete, which causes central nervous system syphilis and has reduced the number of people with paresis (the name of this psychiatric illness) to a very, very low figure in our mental hospitals. But it was a real problem forty years ago. Equally, there is a rare psychosis called pellagra psychosis caused by a specific vitamin deficiency (nicotinic acid), and this is treated very rapidly and effectively by giving this vitamin.

People have claimed that when something straightforward is found, say nicotinic-acid treatment for pellagra psychosis or penicillin for the spirochete that causes paresis, this disease is then ruled out of psychiatry and taken over by internal medicine. In other words when a clear-cut cause of mental illness is found the internists take it over and the psychiatrist is left with the residual disorders, which stay messy and confused. This is not entirely true, as my comments on newer drugs will illustrate. However, we are still pretty much in the position of looking for drugs that have interesting and unusual effects, either on mood and behavior in normal people or on people with psychiatric illness. And it is still pretty much an empirical "chance discovery" rather than a planned search for the cause and for something that will then beneficially affect the disease state produced by the cause.

Historically, it is useful to go back to 1952. At that time in psychiatry drug treatment was of dubious and limited value. Barbiturates were widely used to try to calm disturbed behavior. An agitated, disturbed, schizophrenic patient, who was hearing voices and causing a ruckus on the ward, could be put to sleep with a barbiturate. This would quiet everything down temporarily, but often the patient would wake up slightly more confused and more disturbed than he had been before. It was certainly no long-term solution to the problem. The barbiturates were also given, although reluctantly, to neurotic patients to control anxiety and tension, and without too much evidence of success. Sometimes they were used intravenously as part of psychotherapy, to try to get a patient to remember things that might be causing his illness. This was called narcoanalysis and worked very well in World War II for combat neuroses, particularly combat fatigue, but the technique was not successful in civilian psychiatry. The causes of neuroses in civilians, of course, are more remote and more complex than was usually the case in combat fatigue, in which symptoms were often due to a single severe, overwhelming situation of stress. Further, barbiturates were prescribed with some misgivings because patients used them to attempt suicide and sometimes became psychically and physiologically dependent on (addicted to) them and suffered severe withdrawal symptoms resembling delirium tremens.

Although morphine and scopolamine given together could quiet a disturbed patient temporarily, the combination was not useful for continued treatment because of morphine's addiction potential.

In 1952 electric shock treatment (electroconvulsive treatment) was being used to control disturbed, excited schizophrenic behavior but with only temporary success. It was, however, a useful treatment in patients with severe depression, whose feelings of sadness and/or guilt of pathological intensity would often respond to six or eight convulsive treatments.

Lobotomy, the surgical cutting of certain fibers in the brain, was being tried in chronically hospitalized, severely ill psychiatric patients. Occasionally, some would improve, but by and large the results were unsatisfactory.

Insulin in large doses was used to induce coma in schizophrenic patients with some benefit in some cases, but the treatment was cumbersome, unreliable, expensive to administer, and occasionally dangerous. Even if a series of thirty or forty treatments produced substantial improvement, the durability of this change was uncertain.

Penicillin was quite effective in paresis, a syphilis-caused organic brain syndrome.

Amphetamines (Dexedrine, Methedrine) were being tried in depression, but these stimulant drugs increased the depressed patient's discomfort more frequently than they relieved it. In short, fifteen years ago psychiatry possessed no drug treatments of clear efficacy in the major types of mental illness confronting most psychiatrists. Other treatments were available but were either unpleasant or too drastic. Except for electro-convulsive treatment in depression, they were of modest or unclear therapeutic value.

Since there were no obvious animal models resembling human psychiatric conditions, drug development in the pharmaceutical industry was principally concerned with barbituratelike sedative drugs or amphetaminelike stimulant drugs.

A sedative drug is one that causes relaxation, even to the point of mild drowsiness or sleepiness. Alcohol, for example, can act as a sedative at low doses. A stimulant drug tends to increase alertness, increase activity, and reduce fatigue. Both types of drugs can sometimes cause euphoria, a marked feeling of well-being.*

---

* This drug classification is idealized and based on the more usual effects of the drugs involved. Considerable variability in human response to both classes of drugs can occur, based on differences between individuals and the situation under which the drug is given and the dose taken. A small proportion of people are relaxed by amphetamines, and sedative drugs given in a stimulating environment (*e.g.,* alcohol at a cocktail party) can produce overactive drunken behavior.

In 1952, two new drugs belonging to neither pharmacological class burst onto the psychiatric scene and changed the entire picture. They were chlorpromazine (its trade name is Thorazine) and reserpine (which is marketed under many names). Neither drug was initially used in psychiatric patients and both have interesting histories.

Reserpine was derived from the root of an Indian plant, *Rauwolfia serpentina,* which had been used as a drug by Ayurvedic Hindu naturopaths for centuries. It was found by a modern Indian physician to reduce blood pressure and was tried in the United States as a treatment for hypertension (high blood pressure). Hypertensive patients receiving it were observed to be less anxious and it was then tried in schizophrenic patients by Kline with some success.

Chlorpromazine (Thorazine) was originally synthesized as an antihistamine by a French company. It had unusual effects on the autonomic nervous system. Laborit, in France, used it as part of a drug cocktail designed to reduce the systemic response of patients to surgical injury. These patients were observed to be unusually calm or tranquil after surgery. Acting on this clue, Delay and Deniker tried the drug in disturbed and excited schizophrenic and manic patients and had remarkable success. Rumor has it that a French company, Rhone Poulenc, had offered chlorpromazine to several American firms for promotion and development in the United States before Smith, Kline and French took on the drug, just before its psychiatric use became clear. Given the pharmacological methods then available, none of the other companies were apparently able to detect any worthwhile effects from this new compound. This is noteworthy because this drug and its chemical relatives have had a truly major impact on the treatment of psychiatric patients.

Psychiatry has since gained several other drug types from similarly indirect sources. Meprobamate (Miltown or Equanil) was developed during a search for a muscle-relaxing drug. Iproniazid (Marsalid), the first of one class of new antidepressant drugs, was developed as a treatment for tuberculosis. Imipramine

(Tofranil), the first of our other new major group of antidepressant drugs, was supposed to be a better chlorpromazine. A Swiss psychiatrist (Kuhn) found it did not help schizophrenics but did help patients with depressions.

Many other drugs resembling chlorpromazine or imipramine or meprobamate have been discovered and tested in both animals and man. A fair number of such drugs are in general medical use in this country. Many others are undergoing careful study for both safety and efficacy.

Several reasonable questions may be asked about our present portfolio of psychiatric drugs: What kinds of drugs are there? What are they good for? What limitations do they have? What are their public health or social consequences, if any? What do they teach us about the causes or nature of psychiatric illness?

Existing potent drugs affecting behavior can best be classified into the following groups:

I. *Antipsychotic Drugs*

    A. PHENOTHIAZINES

        (*e.g.,* chlorpromazine [Thorazine], thioridazine, perphenazine, fluphenazine)

    B. RESERPINE

Briefly, these drugs are useful in treating schizophrenia and other psychotic symptoms but in some patients cause neurological side-effects that resemble Parkinson's disease. Chemically the two types of antipsychotic drugs differ greatly, but they are rather similar pharmacologically in several dimensions. Although I believe that the term *antipsychotic* describes these drugs best, they have also been called tranquilizers, a less precise term, which also includes the next group.

II. *Minor Tranquilizers* (*e.g.,* meprobamate [Miltown or Equanil], chlordiazepoxide [Librium], diazepam [Valium])

These drugs as well as chlorpromazine and reserpine were all initially called "tranquilizers" on the assumption that they all relieved anxiety, tension, distress, and fear. It is now clear that the minor tranquilizers do have some effect on anxiety and tension but differ from the antipsychotic drugs described above in lacking any major effect on schizophrenic symptoms such as delusions or hallucinations. There has recently been a revival of interest in the psychiatric use of diphenylhydantoin (Dilantin), a drug used for many years in the treatment of epilepsy. Several preliminary studies suggest the drug may be useful in certain anxiety conditions manifested by irritability and pressure of thought as well as by psychosomatic symptoms. It is too early to say whether this drug is significantly more effective than those otherwise available.

III. *Sedative-Hypnotics* (*e.g.,* barbiturates, Doriden, chloral hydrate, ethchlorvynol [Placidyl])

The differences between these drugs and the minor tranquilizers are a matter of controversy and speculation. Both groups at appropriate dosages can relieve anxiety and produce sedation (sleepiness). All can be used as sleeping pills. Generally, the minor tranquilizers are presumed to relieve more anxiety with less undesirable sedation than the barbiturates. Drugs like meprobamate or chlordiazepoxide are much safer in terms of suicidal danger, since the fatal dose is relatively much larger. Both classes of drugs resemble alcohol in some respects pharmacologically. A patient physically dependent on any of them can probably have his withdrawal symptoms relieved by any of the others unless severe delirium has occurred.

IV. *Opiates* (*e.g.,* morphine, Demerol, codeine)

Drugs like morphine are not usually considered psychiatric drugs because of their addiction liability, that is, their ability to produce both psychological dependence (craving) and physiological dependence manifested by severe withdrawal symptoms. They are generally used in clinical medicine as analgesics to relieve moderate or severe pain. However, in addition to their pain-alleviating actions, they also can reduce anxiety dramatically and can relieve depression or induce euphoria in some individuals. They are clinically used for this purpose before patients go to surgery, and in some patients suffering acute or chronic pain.

V. *Stimulants* (*e.g.,* d-amphetamine [Dexedrine], Methedrine, methylphenidate)

These and related drugs are generally stimulating. They relieve fatigue and counteract impairment in functioning caused by fatigue. Thinking seems speeded and overtalkativeness sometimes occurs. Some people feel pleasantly stimulated, others find the effects unpleasant and react with increased anxiety and tension. These drugs also decrease appetite for food.

VI. *Antidepressants*

These drugs have the property of relieving moderate or severe mood depression in a variety of psychiatric conditions character- ized by abnormal sadness, often accompanied by such symptoms as guilt, hopelessness, concentration difficulty, and insomnia. Two different pharmacological classes have been identified to date, the imipramine-like drugs [*e.g.,* imipramine (Tofranil) and amtriplyline (Elavil)] and the mono-amine oxidase [MAO] inhibitors [*e.g.,* phenelzine (Nardil), tranylcypromine (Par- nate)]. Both classes of drugs act in a slow manner, clinical im- provement in depressed patients most often occurring only after one to three weeks of drug treatment. Improvement, when it occurs, can often result in a complete recovery of the patient from his depressive illness.

VII. *Psychotomimetic Agents* (*e.g.,* LSD, mescaline, psilocybin)

These drugs cause intense, bizarre psychic states characterized by strong, rapidly changing moods—anxiety, depression, elation —changes in the way the world looks and the way one's body feels. Intense memories and feelings may go so far as to produce intense religious or mystical experiences. They may lead to pro- longed or severe psychiatric illnesses. These drugs are currently subject to abuse but may turn out to have some value as an adjunct to psychotherapy in treatment-resistant conditions, such as chronic alcoholism or chronic personality disorders.

THERAPEUTIC USEFULNESS IN PSYCHIATRY

By all odds the most useful and important of these drugs are the antipsychotics. Here the phenothiazines (Thorazine, etc.) are faster acting and more effective than reserpine.

Studies carried out under the psychopharmacology program at the National Institute of Mental Health (NIMH) by grant-supported investigators in a large number of hospitals, as well as studies done by the Veterans Administration and by other investigators, have clearly and repeatedly shown several of the phenothiazines to be substantially better than an inert control substance (placebos or dummy tablets) in the treament of both acute and chronic schizophrenic patients. Our data indicate that these drugs substantially reduce almost all symptoms occurring in the rather heterogeneous group of patients diagnosed as having schizophrenia. Symptoms such as hostility, delusions of persecution, hallucinations and agitation, phenomena which we would call secondary symptoms of the illness, improve considerably. Some improvement in these symptoms is noted in patients acutely ill in the first few hours, but further, gradually increasing benefit is seen for at least three months—longer in some patients. More central primary symptoms—withdrawal from reality, indifference and apathy, deterioration in self-care, bizarre mannerisms—also improve but tend to stop changing earlier, after five or six weeks on the average. As a crude estimate of the power of these drugs in newly hospitalized schizophrenics, the first NIMH multihospital collaborative study showed two-thirds of the phenothiazine-treated patients to be much improved after six weeks of treatment, whereas only a quarter of the placebo-treated patients did as well. Only one-tenth of the phenothiazine-treated patients were unchanged after six weeks, (and none was worse) while half the placebo-treated patients were unchanged or worse, and a third were dropped from the six-week study because they were not doing well.

Chronic schizophrenics show a similar but less dramatic response. The drugs have been shown to help prevent hospitalization in acutely ill patients and to help chronic patients stay out of the hospital for prolonged periods.

Phenothiazines, then, are not fully curative in the sense that penicillin cures pneumonia. Some patients do very well; many others return to, or close to, their pre-illness level of adjustment. Unfortunately this is often rather a borderline and inadequate state of functioning. It may be quite adequate for the patient to remain out of the hospital, but may fall short of full mental health and normal social effectiveness.

These drugs have contributed significantly to the drop in the number of patients in our public mental hospitals, which began in 1955. This drop has continued, as seen on the chart on page 115.

The minor tranquilizers and to a lesser extent the barbiturates are useful in the treatment of anxiety and tension states in neurotic or normal individuals, but are of little use in schizophrenia. Even in neurosis, the evidence from well-controlled large studies is mixed. Drugs such as meprobamate (Miltown or Equanil) or chlordiazepoxide (Librium) generally come out as being a little better than placebo, but not by any dramatic margin. In a series of studies involving three outpatient clinics developed under the NIMH psychopharmacology program to investigate factors that might influence drug and/or placebo response, we have been most struck by the fact that the results differ substantially from clinic to clinic, to the extent that if each clinic were considered as a single study, quite different results would have been reported. What is worse, these differences cannot be accounted for by the known characteristics of the patients treated. Part of the problem may lie in the fact that we have studied new admissions to these clinics. Evidence from other studies shows that patients with anxiety symptoms of recent onset and with little or no previous drug treatment do as well on inert placebo as on drugs, 80 per cent of patients improving under either treatment. Patients with chronic symptoms and more previous exposure to drugs do substantially

Projected and Actual Numbers of Resident Patients
End of Year in State and County Mental Hospitals—United States—1946–1966

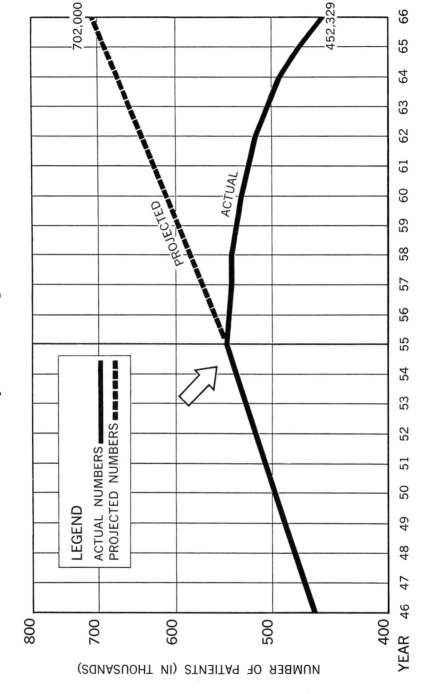

better on drugs than on placebo; 80 per cent improve on drugs as against 25 per cent on placebo.

We also have some evidence that these drugs may show their power more by changing a patient's attitude to his environment than by reducing his symptoms. Patients on chlordiazepoxide [Librium], for example, describe their doctor as a nicer person than do patients on placebo, and patients on this drug reported that more "good" things happened to them while under treatment than did patients on placebo. The "good" things, interestingly, sounded generally as though the patients were more aggressive and were pleased by it. They described vigorous discussions of mutual problems with their employer or their spouse as "good" events.

This all fits with one pharmacological theory of the differences between the minor tranquilizers and the phenothiazines (Mellaril, Thorazine, etc.) in the treatment of anxiety. In animals, and apparently in man, the minor tranquilizers may reduce anxiety and increase activity and adventurousness. Under the influence of these drugs animals will risk a painful shock to get something they want. Without the drug they won't take the risk. In man this could be viewed as the drug decreasing inhibitions. These drugs may also increase response to the environment. The phenothiazines, on the other hand, reduce anxiety but increase inhibitions and permit the animal or the patient to ignore some aspects of his environment. Activity may be reduced somewhat.

The stimulants—amphetamine [Dexedrine] or Ritalin—have little use in adult psychiatry. Occasional patients with chronic fatigue or mild depression may do well on them but in at least one controlled study mildly depressed patients improved more on inert placebo than they did on amphetamine. When taken to excess illicitly, these drugs can produce a severe psychotic episode strikingly similar to paranoid schizophrenia, usually marked by intense fear and delusions of persecution by the police or Communists or the FBI.

The stimulant drugs have one unique clinical use, however. In children who present a hyperkinetic behavior disorder marked by restless, scattered overactivity, very short attention span, and poor school performance, these drugs frequently substantially improve the child, allowing him to apply himself to his school work and control and focus his energies in a healthier manner. The reasons for this are not clear, but these drugs act more like a tranquilizer than a stimulant in such children; barbiturate sedatives usually make them worse.

The antidepressants of both the MAO (such as Nardil and Parnate) and imipramine types (such as Elavil and Tofranil) pose a problem. These drugs generally appear less effective in carefully controlled clinical studies than the experience of senior clinical psychiatrists would suggest. In controlled studies the drugs are usually shown to be better than placebo, but not dramatically so. Clinicians report generally more favorable results in ordinary clinical use. From the literature it looks as though six or seven out of ten patients might do well on imipramine, while four or five out of ten would do well on inert placebo. The MAO inhibitors generally look a bit less effective than the imipramine-like drugs. The NIMH is currently supporting and coordinating a ten-hospital collaborative study to determine what kinds of depressed patients need what drug and what kinds of patients do quite well on placebo alone. The results of treatment on imipramine and an antipsychotic phenothiazine are now being analyzed, and a study of an MAO inhibitor and a minor tranquilizer is now under way. Some drugs not classified as antidepressants, both antipsychotics and minor tranquilizers, are reported to help some depressed patients.

The literature suggests that patients with severe retarded (slowed and inhibited) depressions do best on imipramine, whereas anxious patients with less severe depressions may do as well or better on a phenothiazine. Some patients who fail to respond to an imipramine-like drug do well on an MAO inhibitor. The final status of all this is far from clear. Electroconvulsive therapy is still the most reliable treatment for severe depression.

It is now probably safer and less unpleasant since patients are usually anesthetized before the treatment and given a muscle-relaxing drug to reduce the physical stress of the convulsion. Prolonged medication with antidepressant drugs may help prevent the recurrence of depression in patients who have had a series of such illnesses. The new antidepressant drugs have opened many interesting leads in research on the abnormal biochemistry of depressed patients.

Psychotomimetic drugs, chiefly LSD, are currently being studied as part of psychotherapy programs in the treatment of chronic alcoholics, chronic neurotics and patients with chronic personality disorders. Patients often show an initially positive enthusiastic response to this treatment, and several controlled studies in this general area are now under way under NIMH grant support to determine whether these effects have any lasting value. Preliminary results look promising, although there is some suggestion that treatment-induced positive changes may begin to fade after six months or so.

In addition to the above knowledge—complete and partial—about older drugs, newer things are appearing on the horizon. Although some of the newer drugs being developed by the pharmaceutical industry appear unfortunately similar to existing drugs, some give hints of more promise. Several newer antipsychotic drugs may turn out to control symptoms as well as do the phenothiazines but may give chronic schizophrenic patients more energy and drive and enable them to cope more effectively with the real world outside hospitals. The search for a more effective and faster-acting antidepression drug is ongoing. Current studies—which suggest that depressed patients have a deficiency in noradrenalin, show abnormally overactive adrenal cortices, and have abnormalities in the balance of electrolytes (sodium and potassium) inside and outside their cells—may lead the way to a specific drug treatment designed to correct these abnormalities.

A growing number of experimental drugs are emerging, which

appear to have specific effects on the production or destruction of a variety of important brain chemicals and may lead first to firmer knowledge of the chemical bases of behavior and later to better, more rational drug treatments.

In another area, an electrolyte, lithium, appears to have a specific effect in controlling manic excitements—states characterized by severe and excessive happiness, overactivity, grandiosity, and bad judgment—and in preventing the recurrence of such states. Recent European data suggest that lithium may also prevent the recurrence of depression, even though it has no effect on depression once the illness is present.

Cyclazocine, a drug that can completely block the effects of heroin or morphine, is showing promise in the treatment of heroin addiction. If such patients take cyclazocine daily, they are prevented, almost completely, from getting any "kicks" out of illicit heroin and are therefore not tempted to resume their addiction to this drug.

An old antiepileptic drug, diphenylhydantoin, either alone or in combination with one of the phenothiazines, is reported to help severe behavior disorders in adolescents or young adults who show impulsive disruptive semidelinquent behavior.

The drug industry is actively looking for drugs that will improve memory. The most publicized of these, magnesium pemmoline (Cylert), although interesting in animal studies, appears to be less active in clinical studies. Other drugs of this sort are almost certain to follow.

The NIMH, which recently was elevated to Bureau status within the Public Health Service, has an active program for studying and evaluating drug treatments in psychiatry and has been quite successful in getting needed clinical studies of clearly promising drugs carried out. It also supports a number of research units devoted to finding out what very new drugs may be able to do in treating a variety of psychiatric conditions. Also supported is research that investigates the mechanisms by which these drugs act as well as more basic aspects of brain function and its relationship to behavior. Information on new research development in psychopharmacology is provided to investigators in this field through two publications of NIMH's National Clearinghouse for Mental Health Information, *Psychopharmacology Abstracts* and the *Psychopharmacology Bulletin.*

As one looks back at the drug treatments coming into psychiatry in the past fifteen years, what can one say about their impact? They have certainly helped speed the release of patients from psychiatric hospitals or psychiatric wards in general hospitals and have helped reduce the number of patients in public mental hospitals in the face of an ever-growing number of patient admissions. If the number of hospitalized patients had continued to grow at the pre-1955 rate, about two billion dollars more would have been spent on hospitalization costs alone, excluding the costs of building many new facilities to house a growing mass of patients. Losses in earning power on the part of these patients are also not included in this figure.

It is also reasonable to assume that drug treatments have speeded and eased the development of new and improved patterns of treatment for the mentally ill and emotionally disturbed. Examples are day-care centers, sheltered workshops, and community mental health centers, which hopefully will incorporate all appropriate levels and patterns of psychiatric care. The drugs also assist physicians who are not psychiatrists in handling psychiatric problems. Since it is currently unlikely that this country can train enough psychiatrists to meet all needs, the ability of general practitioners and internists to function effectively in this area is highly desirable.

The liabilities of these drugs, though present, are quite small by comparison. Some of the drugs, particularly the phenothiazines and antidepressants, can cause mildly disagreeable side effects—drowsiness, dry mouth, nausea, tremors, and skin rashes —that are usually not difficult to manage or are tolerable. More severe toxic effects—blood-cell depression, convulsions, serious liver abnormalities—are fortunately quite rare. Fatalities attributable to these drugs are very, very rare indeed.

Abuse of the older drugs—barbiturates, opiates, and stimulants—has existed for many years in unstable individuals. The phenothiazines and antidepressants appear almost totally without abuse liability; their effects on subjective mood are generally not initially pleasurable. The minor tranquilizers and nonbarbiturate sedatives can be abused, but so far this abuse appears minor. They are not usually sold illicitly. The few patients who have developed physical dependence on them—this usually occurs when more than ten to fifteen pills are taken daily—seem to have obtained their excessive supply of pills from one or more unwary physicians.

It has been feared that these drugs might interfere with psychotherapy. There is no real evidence that this occurs. In a few studies involving schizophrenic patients, drugs are clearly superior to psychotherapy alone, while drugs plus psychotherapy show slight superiority to drugs alone.

There is an ethical, almost religious, but also practical question that has never really been studied because it presents very large administrative-logistic problems. It pertains chiefly to the minor antianxiety drugs. It is: Should people suffer out the anxiety of life and solve their problems or should the anxiety be relieved by drugs? If it is, do problems go unsolved? A similar problem is: Suppose a drug makes the patient feel better—who is responsible for making sure he isn't behaving worse, at least in the eyes of his family or his employer? These things have never been thoroughly investigated, although one group of workers evaluating the effects of a minor tranquilizer found that both the patients and their relatives judged the drug effects to be more positive in areas of social functioning and generally saw more improvement than did the treating physicians. All one can say after at least ten years' experience with minor tranquilizers is that more complaints would have been voiced loudly on many occasions if these problems were major ones. At least one hopes this is the case.

Another worry is sometimes voiced that drugs will be developed that will control the mind and permit mass brainwashing.

For the near future, at least, this worry seems completely unfounded. Laboratory, clinical, and research workers are having considerable trouble developing better drugs to control rather gross abnormalities, like depression or chronic alcoholism, and interesting new drug types continue to emerge as much by chance as by rational procedures. The odds of finding drugs that control more discrete thoughts or attitudes in normal citizens seem awfully small and well outside current technology.

It also has been often hoped that the new drugs will help us find the biological causes of mental illnesses. Two points are worth mentioning here:

1. Even if a drug corrects an abnormal state of functioning, this does not mean that the abnormal state was caused by a biochemical defect. If a biological or biochemical abnormality is being corrected by a drug, the abnormality could still have been produced by a psychological or social stress.

2. At the moment the drugs, and other newer agents, are teaching us a great deal about how the normal brain works and are giving valuable leads about abnormalities related to severe depression or manic elation. The relevance to schizophrenia, that is to the abnormal processes underlying schizophrenia, is less clear.

Until recently, in fact, a paradox existed. Two drug classes—the reserpinelike drugs and the MAO inhibitors—had clear and dramatic effects on brain biochemistry, but were not very useful clinically, whereas the phenothiazines and the imipramine-type antidepressants appeared to be effective therapeutically, but had no obvious biochemical effects. Recently, interesting but more subtle biochemical effects have been found for these more potent drugs.

One aspect of the newer psychiatric drugs, separable from the scientific and clinical evidence about their effectiveness, is the magnitude of their use in the United States. A recent scientific national population survey carried out by Cisin and Cahalan of George Washington University showed that 18 per cent of the adult women and 9 per cent of the men in this country admitted finding tranquilizers helpful when they felt "depressed or nervous." An even larger proportion (29 per cent of the women and 17 per cent of the men) admitted finding "other pills or medicines" helpful under the same circumstances.

Data from a national survey of prescriptions filled by drugstores disclosed that 16 per cent of all prescriptions were for psychiatric drugs. In general these drugs seem to be prescribed more for women than for men and more for people of middle age or older than for young adults. The Cisin and Cahalan survey noted above was specifically directed toward alcohol-drinking practices. These same investigators are now developing, under grant support, a national survey aimed at understanding the patterns and extent of psychoactive drug use, the reasons underlying such use, and the social and psychological characteristics of people taking such drugs.

Presently available data can only tell us that drugs are rather widely used for psychiatric or emotional disorders or symptoms. It is impossible to place any valid value judgment on such data, although alarmists can claim too much use and enthusiasts can claim that more, or more appropriate, use is highly desirable.

During a recent study of drug efficacy in chronic schizophrenia, we obtained data indicating that 90 per cent of such patients were currently receiving drug treatment. Informal figures from private psychiatric hospitals, even those emphasizing psychotherapy as the major treatment approach, suggest that at least 40 per cent of more acutely ill patients receive drugs, while figures from public hospitals would be much higher.

It is clear that the drugs are widely used and often useful, but it is equally clear that for many individual patients, and for some large patient groups (*e.g.,* chronic alcoholics), much better drug treatments are needed.

In summary, several useful classes of new psychiatric drugs have emerged in the last fifteen years. They have had a major impact on psychiatric treatment and basic research. Their full consequences are not yet finally evident. Hopefully, the future will yield even more powerful and useful agents.

NOTE ON CONTRIBUTOR

Jonathan O. Cole (M.D., 1947, Cornell Medical College) is currently superintendent, Boston State Hospital, and professor of psychiatry, Tufts University School of Medicine. At the time of this presentation, he was chief of psychopharmacology, Research Branch, National Institute of Mental Health, Bethesda, Maryland, and associate clinical professor of psychiatry, Georgetown University, Washington, D.C. He was president of the American College of Neuropsychopharmacology in 1966 and presently is American secretary to the Collegium Internationale Neuro-Psychopharmacologicum and a member of the National Academy of Sciences, National Research Council committee on problems of drug dependence. He is a member of the editorial board of the *American Journal of Psychiatry* and a fellow of the American Association for the Advancement of Science and of the American Orthopsychiatric Association.

7

Experimental Design of Anticancer Agents

MORRIS E. FRIEDKIN, PH.D.

NOTWITHSTANDING A MASSIVE worldwide research effort maintained now for several decades, the cancers, except for two rare forms, are generally incurable by drug treatment alone.

Why then do many medical scientists remain hopeful for a successful chemical treatment of cancer?

Despite the likelihood that the immunization techniques so useful in many diseases caused by germs and viruses may be applied eventually for the prevention and cure of certain cancers, the drug-kill of cancer cells remains an important objective of cancer research. Many types of cancer are indeed partially responsive to drugs. A special reason for hope is that choriocarcinoma, a most malignant and disseminated form of cancer, once an inevitably fatal disease, has been cured with drugs. "If choriocarcinoma (a type of cancer that arises from the placenta during or after pregnancy) can respond most favorably to chemical treatment, why not similar successes in the more common forms of cancer?" medical scientists ask.

Perhaps if properly used, many of the agents now available

could be more effective. This concept of re-examining in depth how we could make better use of presently available drugs represents a major effort in the highly organized area of controlled studies of drug efficacy in cancer patients.

The vocabulary of war has been taken over by scientists in the "battle to conquer" the cancers. At the National Cancer Institute areas of intensive research are being mapped for attack by the Acute Leukemia Task Force, the Lymphoma Task Force, the Chronic Leukemia and Multiple Myeloma Task Force, and the Breast Cancer Task Force. The purpose of the *task force* is to coordinate major research tactics for better control of a particular form of cancer.

This approach has led, for example, to promising new drug schedules in the treatment of acute leukemia of childhood. More about this later.

But no matter how well organized or aggressive a program for cancer research, no matter how promising the final solutions, the hope of many patients with cancer must rest with drugs of tomorrow, and unfortunately, not with those of today.

This may be a pessimistic outlook, but the statistics for five-year cancer survival rates for selected sites of cancer, such as lung and stomach, are not encouraging.

The initial area where the malignant process arises may be detected early and is referred to as "localized." If detection is delayed and the cancer becomes more generally dispersed, it is referred to as "regional." It is obvious that early detection and diagnosis of cancer are reflected by a much better chance for five-year survival.

For example, in breast cancer early detection and treatment of a localized malignancy there is an 82 per cent five-year survival rate, whereas late detection cuts the survival rate to 46 per cent. In stomach cancer a 40 per cent survival rate is obtained upon early detection, whereas regional involvement drops the rate to 12 per cent. Figures for lung cancer are the least encouraging with only 21 per cent survival even with early detection, and the discouraging low value of only 5 per cent with regional involvement.

The impact of cancer is staggering. About one out of every four people alive in the United States today can be expected to develop cancer at some time during his or her lifetime. With a

AREA	% 5 YR. SURVIVAL	
	LOCALIZED	REGIONAL
SKIN	92	——
BREAST	82	46
BLADDER	68	24
PROSTATE	50	30
STOMACH	40	12
LUNG	21	5

growing population and an increasing proportion of older persons, deaths due to cancer will continue to rise in the next decade. By 1975 there will be more than a million cancer cases under treatment each year, with an annual death toll of 300,000. An even more somber projection is based on the alarming increase in lung cancer, a disease characterized, as I have just indicated, by a very high mortality even with early detection. Aside from the immeasurable cost in human suffering, the economic burden of cancer is more than twelve billion dollars a year in the United States.

For patients with disseminated cancer, a situation in which surgery and radiation are ineffective, the only hope is an agent that can be carried by the blood stream to all parts of the body, to poison the malignant cells, wherever they may reside, without harming the normal cells.

How then can new drugs best be discovered or designed, modified, and developed for therapeutic effect in cancer?

Biochemists and pharmacologists in the field of cancer chemotherapy are deeply concerned about the design of new agents. Cancer research is costly. With millions of dollars spent already and with cures always just around the corner despite the most promising preliminary results, the medical scientist must constantly reappraise his strategy in the chemical assault against the cancers.

THE CANCER PROBLEM

How do you go about ridding the body of cancer cells that begin to divide and spread, unrestrained by the usual controls of the body?

The cancer cell is not unusual in its ability to divide. Within us are many normal cell types that divide again and again *but always* under the most sensitive control.

For example, as our red blood cells gradually age and become more fragile, they are more apt to burst. This is a natural decay process, which would inexorably deplete the blood stream of red cells unless replenished by young cells from the bone marrow. Within our bone marrow are primitive cells, dividing constantly, maturing, and finally delivering into the blood stream a new source of red cells. There are also rapidly dividing cells in the lining of the intestine. These cells, too, are under good control.

The malignant cancer cell, on the other hand, has escaped the controls of the body. It not only keeps dividing, but also, like a weed, scatters throughout the body.

Well, how do you weed a lawn without destroying the grass? Either by hand, or in recent years with amazing weed poisons. Consider the selective process that accomplishes the weeding. In one case the gardener with a keen eye recognizes crabgrass, dandelion, or chickweed, and cuts out these weeds by hand. In the other case the agricultural chemist has taken advantage of the broad-leafed shape of the weeds. When a lawn is sprayed with a weedkiller, the broad-leafed weeds pick up a higher concentration of the poison than the relatively narrow-bladed bluegrass.

A similar kind of recognition is necessary in "weeding" the body of cancer cells. The pathologist recognizes the mosaiclike quality of a patch of cancer cells. This recognition guides the surgeon who removes, "weeds out," the malignant cells. But when the weeds are widespread, handcutting becomes impossible. How, then, can the art of the chemical weed-killer be applied to cancer?

Any strategy aimed at wiping out a population of malignant cells by chemical means must take into account the implications of unrestrained cell reproduction by the process of doubling. The reproduction of a single malignant cell, upon doubling within a twenty-four-hour period, increases the population by one cell. The increase in population when a million cells double is many magnitudes higher, amounting to a million cells within the same time span of twenty-four hours.

As a result of exponential increase, a single leukemic cell, when transplanted to a mouse, can give rise within three weeks to over a billion malignant cells. It has been estimated that the average eight-year-old, sixty-six-pound child with acute leukemia may have as many as a trillion (10^{12}) leukemic cells in his body.

It follows, therefore, that if acute leukemia is to be curable, the drug must successfully wipe out all of these cells. The escape of only a few cells leads inevitably to an astronomical increase of progeny.

The problem of drug therapy is made even more complicated by factors such as drug resistance and limitations to the general distribution of the agent within the body. Cells once vulnerable to drug attack can build up resistance so that an initially effective dose loses its punch. By the genetic process of mutation, cells may become inherently resistant to a drug. Furthermore, cells may escape drug action by growing in the sanctuary of the brain, where most of the effective antileukemic agents cannot penetrate.

Another vexing problem in drug therapy of cancer is the absence of a normal immunological reaction of the body to the malignant cells. In most infections that are successfully combatted by use of antibiotics, it is not an absolute requirement that each germ be eradicated by direct action of the antibiotic. Since the human body recognizes the invading organism as foreign, specific antibodies are elaborated as a defense mechanism to neutralize the cells that may have escaped the action of an antibiotic such as penicillin or streptomycin. Parenthetically, it is quite possible that drug cures in choriocarcinoma and in the Burkitt lymphoma in African children may be attributable in part to an immune response by the patient.

Unfortunately, most cancer cells are not recognized by the body as foreign. Furthermore, most drugs used as anticancer agents may actually interfere with the immune mechanism. As a consequence, cancer cells can multiply to a fantastic degree without any apparent immunological response, that is no defensive elaboration of antibodies to the malignant cell. The implication of this is that drug therapy must be completely effective for a cure. A percentage of 99.99 is not good enough. For if only 0.01 per cent of one million cells survive after drug treatment, this is equivalent to one hundred cells, which by exponential increase can go on to repopulate with fatal consequences.

For these reasons new schedules of drug therapy have been developed with the aim of achieving a virtually complete eradication of a cell population. Such schedules combine at least four drugs, each of which has a different mechanism of killing action.

Designated the VAMP program, each letter stands for a different therapeutic agent: V for vincristine, A for amethopterin, M for 6-mercaptopurine, and P for prednisone. This new approach of intensive drug therapy has raised new hope for more effective treatment of acute leukemia, a disease that kills about 2,100 children a year in the United States. Since the introduction of antifolic compounds by Dr. Sidney Farber in Boston twenty years ago, the median survival of children with acute leukemia has been increased from about four months to fourteen months. Within the next two or three years we should have enough data to evaluate the effectiveness of the VAMP program.

Having discussed some of the main problems we face in developing effective anticancer agents, I would now like to turn to the key question of this discussion: How does one design new anticancer drugs?

One approach is to look at those drugs now in use, to proceed by analogy, and hopefully to profit by experience. Let us consider a few examples.

NITROGEN MUSTARD

Out of man's incessant quest for more efficient means to kill and to maim his enemy came mustard gas, first used by the Germans in July of 1917 in the bombardment of British positions in Flanders. The effects were devastating. One of the serious poisoning effects of mustard gas was seen as a decrease in the number of white blood cells, a fact seized upon years later by medical scientists to combat diseases in which there is an unrestrained growth of certain white cells.

Between World Wars I and II work continued on chemical warfare agents, resulting in the synthesis of a modified form of mustard gas, *i.e.,* nitrogen mustard. Within a framework of military secrecy, extensive clinical studies were carried out with the classified chemical warfare agents during World War II. Thus a new class of valuable chemo-therapeutic drugs, the nitrogen mustards, has emerged as a result of man's inhumanity to man.

The lesson for us in this is: An agent toxic to man (*i.e.,* cytotoxic) may also be toxic to his cancer cells. With chemical modification the agent can be designed to be more toxic toward the cancer cell than toward man.

In more general terms, a cytotoxic agent that poisons a living

$$S \diagup^{CH_2 \quad CH_2 \quad Cl}_{\diagdown \, CH_2 \quad CH_2 \quad Cl}$$

MUSTARD GAS

(used to kill)

$$CH_3 - N \diagup^{CH_2 \quad CH_2 \quad Cl}_{\diagdown \, CH_2 \quad CH_2 \quad Cl}$$

NITROGEN MUSTARD

(used in chemotherapy)

cell—be it from a man or a mouse, a plant or a bacterium—has the potential of being an anticancer agent, if chemically modified into a form that is less dangerous to man. Unfortunately, in most cases anticancer agents are very toxic. In many situations of cancer chemotherapy, when drug therapy is pushed to the extreme, drug toxicity is as threatening to life as the cancer process itself.

In fact, in certain cases drugs not only eradicate cancer cells, but also wipe out the white cells that are so essential in warding off infection. For this reason, complex supportive therapy must accompany the cancer drug therapy so as to help the patient survive the toxic effects of the cancer drug. Antibiotics, sterile surroundings, and special platelet and white cell transfusions are often required.

HORMONAL CONTROL OF CANCER

In 1939 Dr. Charles Huggins and his associates at the University of Chicago reported that the integrity and function of the prostate gland is dependent on a constant source of male sex hormone (androgen) and that the administration of female sex hormone (estrogen) can block the effects of the androgen. Dr. Huggins postulated that if in advanced prostatic carcinoma the malignant cells are still dependent on male sex hormone for continued proliferation, then removal of the source of androgen and treatment with estrogen should lead to a significant clinical improvement. This theory proved to be correct, leading to one of the safest forms of cancer chemotherapy, the clinical use of either natural or synthetic forms of female sex hormone in the treatment of cancer of the prostrate.

Dr. Huggins was recently honored for his role in the development of successful androgen-control procedures; in 1966, twenty-five years after he first proposed this rational approach, he was awarded the Nobel Prize.

Again this holds an important lesson: Perhaps in other neoplastic diseases malignant cells may be dependent on hormones for continued growth. Either by cutting off the supply of natural hormone or by interfering with hormonal action, control of the cancer process should be possible. Indeed, estrogens and androgens have been found to be useful in the treatment of breast cancer, especially when the lesions are too widespread to permit effective surgery or radiation.

One of the main difficulties with this approach is that cancer cells, initially requiring hormonal activation, may progressively lose their dependence by gradually changing into malignant cell types that can grow in the absence of hormone.

THE VINCA ALKALOIDS

For many years the periwinkle plant (*Vinca rosea*) has had a folklore reputation as a "cure-all." In Brazil, an extract of the leaves was supposed to be good for scurvy, bleeding, and for toothaches; in British West Indies, for ulcers; and in the Philippines, South Africa, and England, for diabetes. Because of its reputed effect as an insulin substitute, the periwinkle plant became the subject of intense research by two groups of investigators in Canada and the United States. As a substitute for insulin it was found to be useless. However, the Canadian group observed that certain fractions from the plant decreased the white count in the blood of experimental rats and that a toxic effect on the bone marrow was produced. At about the same time the American group found that certain fractions from the leaves would prolong the lifespan of mice implanted with leukemic cells. This was considered a significant finding since the same tumor system had been used to detect other clinically useful antitumor agents. As a result of these findings, vincristine, a basic substance of the plant, is now being used in the treatment of acute leukemia.

In regard to this, there is yet another lesson: There are all kinds of unknown substances in nature that might have anticancer activity. Set up a screen with an experimental tumor, grown either in animals or in tissue culture, and test thousands upon thousands of extracts from plants, fungi, insects, marine life, and fermented brews. Strike into the jungle and collect! Keep an ear open for any kind of witchcraft, any old wives' tale, any folklore, and test indiscriminately just as Edison did when he was looking for the right kind of long-burning filament in his electric light.

A good example of the continuing search for naturally occurring medicinal agents is the subject of a newspaper account in *The New York Times* of January 22, 1967 (see headline on opposite page). For many years a popular medicine of the inhabitants of the north coast of Honduras has been a crude tea brewed from a fern that grows as a parasite on the palm tree.

The article reports that an extract of the fern has produced encouraging preliminary results in inhibiting the growth of cancer cells, and that "striking" improvement in terminal cancer patients was seen. The reporter, knowing the elements of a good story, informs the reader that the fern was shipped from a region named

A HONDURAN FERN TESTED IN CANCER

Extract of a Palm Parasite Appears to Inhibit Cells

Gracia a Dios (Thanks to God)! Later on I will say more about premature disclosure of information about presumably effective anticancer agents.

During the last ten years a total of 257,000 materials have been screened in an enormous test program set up by the National Cancer Institute. The actual experimental work has been carried out in laboratories of universities, industry, and governmental facilities. The cost of this empirical work has been very high. Must we continue to employ such empirical methods, making giant sweeps through the underbrush of the world in search of new anticancer agents?

The question really is one of the rational approach versus empirical research. An enormous fountain of new information about cell biology has erupted during the last decade. Molecular biology, a new discipline, has revealed much about how genetic information is stored within chromosomes and how the chemical blueprint for cell growth and cell function is "read." These exciting discoveries are all in the language of biochemistry, with complex chemical structures that are difficult to interpret to the non-biochemist. Just as the space program has generated a lively language of its own, molecular biology spawns such jargon as the *triplet code, repressor, allosteric system, operon, regulator genes, transfer RNA, information transfer,* and *messenger RNA.*

Do these exciting new discoveries in molecular biology have any immediate practical implications in the chemical control of cancer? I believe that the average citizen too often is misled by accounts of "promising breakthroughs" in basic research. The development of new drugs based on fundamental concepts of molecular biology, unfortunately, cannot occur overnight. Years of intensive effort are required.

We have come a long way in understanding the intricate biochemical and biophysical events and catalysts of the living cell; yet the living cell, a product of billions of years of evolution, will not spill out all of its secrets within this century.

I firmly believe that a basic knowledge of cell biology is required to understand why cells become malignant, and with this understanding will come a means of blocking the process of malignancy. Many cancer cells exhibit abnormal chromosomes upon microscopic examination. Numerous studies now underway are concerned with the possible relationship between the transformation of a healthy cell into a cancerous one and the basic genetic determinant within the chromosomes: deoxyribonucleic acid, commonly referred to as DNA.

Many factors can operate to influence the DNA of a normal cell. It is a reasonable hypothesis that carcinogens, *i.e.,* chemicals that cause cancer, may produce abnormalities or irreversible changes in the DNA. It is well known that various forms of radiation (ultraviolet light, X-ray, emissions from radioisotopes) can initiate the cancerous change, again by a mechanism that involves changes in the DNA.

If a virus can be shown to induce cancer in man—a phenomenon amply demonstrated in animals—then the interaction between the genetic apparatus of the virus and that of the healthy cell it infects becomes a matter of critical concern. In fact carcinogenesis, the origin of cancer, may depend in part on the activation of latent viruses in healthy tissue. In other words pre-existing viruses in normal cells may remain dormant for many years, to be awakened by some irritant or change in the cellular environment.

What I have just described is an active and important area of research for which there are no assured short-term answers. Any premature promise in this regard is cruel to the cancer patient who requires immediate help. But in the immediate future there are things that can be done with the knowledge at hand. This, I believe, involves a mixture of rational and empirical approaches.

We know much about the biochemistry of normal and cancer cells. Although some biochemical differences exist, it is the unfortunate over-all similarity of the normal and cancer cell that has defeated most attempts to fashion specific poisons for the malignant cells. All dividing cells are critically dependent on certain key reactions, such as the conversion of chemical energy into a useful form for the synthesis of cellular units, or the reactions involved in the copying of genetic units of the cell, or the on-off switching reactions that maintain a proper balance of the myriad chemical events that continue as long as the cell is alive. All of these functions are subject to poisoning by chemical substances modified in structure so as to interfere with basic cell function.

We can make important use of this knowledge. Learn the biochemistry of the cell, *i.e.,* the shape of the keys that turn on and turn off a number of critical reactions within the cell. Make new keys with just enough distortion to jam important locks of the malignant cell but not those of the normal cells. This approach combines both elements of an "educated guess" about the proper chemical conformation of a useful drug and empirical screening. I believe it is to be preferred over indiscriminate screening of any compound off the shelf.

I would like to present three examples of the use of *anti-metabolites*. These are drugs that resemble important chemicals of the body machinery but interfere with the normal mechanisms of cell function. Amethopterin, an analogue of folic acid, is used in the treatment of acute leukemia in children and in a highly malignant cancer in women, choriocarcinoma.

FOLIC ACID — A vitamin

AMETHOPTERIN used in chemotherapy

The purine analogue of hypoxanthine, 6-mercaptopurine, is also used in the treatment of acute leukemia in children (see diagram on page 139).

The pyrimidine analogue of uracil, 5-fluorouracil, has a palliative effect in certain types of advanced carcinoma of the breast and of the gastrointestinal tract (see diagram on page 140).

Even in cases where a normal and malignant cell share equally

HYPOXANTHINE
a building block of the cell

6−MERCAPTOPURINE
used in chemotherapy

sensitive key reactions, thus making it apparently impossible to separate toxicity from therapeutic efficacy, advantage can be taken of differential permeability, the ability of a drug to pass through the cell wall. This approach is worthy of more intensive investigation.

Let us return briefly to the emotional element in the reporting of cancer research. The word "cancer" strikes fear because the public knows that cancer is difficult to treat. It is not surprising, therefore, that the reader of newspapers and magazines is all too ready to accept the latest panacea, be it a new wonder serum or a new nature diet.

At a meeting held specifically to consider the best means whereby the public can learn about medical advances, Dennis Flanagan, Editor of *Scientific American,* said:

I absolutely wince when I think of how many stories I have read (and some I have written myself) about drugs and procedures which show some promise in cancer. I need hardly tell you how few bear out any promise. Taking advantage of hindsight, I am quite sure it would have been better if most of these stories had not been published at all. . . . At worst such stories can give false hope and cause much emotional suffering.

URACIL – a building block   5–FLUOROURACIL
         of the cell   used in chemotherapy

Now let us look at a recent newspaper headline:

CANCER VACCINE TESTED SECRETLY

Controversial Drug Is Given 100 Patients in Cleveland

Here is a classic example of the sensational cancer story, the type still receiving extended coverage by some news media. (Fortunately, many major newspapers today are exercising more responsibility and have medical reporters who do a careful and creditable job.)

The story first broke on page one of the Cleveland *Plain Dealer* on August 19, 1966, when the newspaper's *financial editor* reported that "a cure of cancer long hoped for, may be imminent"; and that rumors of the successful treatment had initiated a scramble for the common stock of the company involved in the development of the cancer vaccine. Wide publicity followed in a nationally circulated magazine, its cover reading: "At last! Scientists report anticancer vaccine. Claim 12 dying patients saved in first experiments!" This "claim" helped to start a pilgrimage of terminal cancer patients to Cleveland. For instance, this article lists Sheik Mahomet Ali, 61, of Pakistan as one of the patients being treated with the new vaccine.

As is often the case with miracle drugs, the inference is made that the forces of conservative medicine and the United States Government regularly conspire to stifle any imaginative approach to the cure for cancer. For example, a headline in *The New York Times* (February 17, 1967) informs the reader that: "U.S. Seeks to Ban a Cancer Vaccine." This in reference to the Cleveland vaccine.

The government seeks to control the use of the Cleveland vaccine, because by law the Food and Drug Administration has the responsibility for ensuring the safety of drugs. Any drug in general use must be proven safe as well as effective in well-controlled clinical studies.

Some years ago, Alfred North Whitehead wrote:

There are no whole truths. All truths are half-truths. It is trying to treat them as whole truths that plays the devil.

I think this admonition is particularly appropriate in the case of the Cleveland vaccine.

It is true, of course, that cancer immunology *is* an expanding

area of cancer research. Much effort is now going into a study of
the possibility that anticancer defenses of cancer patients can be
stimulated by use of vaccines made from cancer tissue: an attempt to make cancer cells subject to control by immune mechanisms. The pity of it is that the efficacy of a new drug or vaccine
cannot be adequately evaluated in an atmosphere charged with
controversial claims and counterclaims.

One of the most common experiences of medicine is referred
to as the "placebo effect." When a patient has confidence in his
doctor and the doctor says, "Take this medicine three times a
day," the patient may show an amazing response for a while, even
though the capsule may contain only sugar. I am not saying that
the currently controversial Cleveland vaccine is a hoax, a mixture
of sugar and oil, so to speak. I am asserting, however, that a
terminal cancer patient with new hope will undoubtedly show
some subjective improvement upon receiving a reputedly effective
anticancer agent—a classic example of the placebo effect.

There are well-known methods of overcoming bias in the evaluation of new drugs—and vaccines. Each must gain scientific
documentation. When clinical trials are carefully performed, five-
year survival rates eventually reveal the true story.

We now face an extraordinary situation in which the ordinary
citizen is either forced to breathe polluted air containing known
carcinogenic substances; or else, by habit, he gambles with his
health by chronic inhalation of smoke proven to be carcinogenic.
The problem of protecting the population from carcinogens is
beyond the scope of this presentation.

The concept of viruses as a cause of cancer has generated
much excitement recently. In the past two years Congress has
appropriated $27,000,000 specifically for virus-leukemia re-
search.

Actually the relationship of virus to cancer goes back many
years. Fifty-five years ago Dr. Peyton Rous described a virus that
causes the transmission of a type of cancer in chickens, named
the Rous chicken sarcoma virus. Last year Dr. Rous was

awarded the Nobel Prize in belated recognition of his fundamental discovery.

The major events in the development of the field of cancer
virology have been reviewed recently by Dr. Eugene Day, who
analyzed the reasons for past skepticism concerning viruses as
causative agents in cancer. For many years there were many who
believed that the Rous chicken sarcoma virus was nothing more
than a chemical carcinogen. There were others who accepted the
fact that a virus was involved, but maintained nevertheless that
findings in chicken cancer were not applicable to animal cancer,
including types afflicting humans.

However, during the last fifteen years much pertinent information about cancer virology has accumulated. In mouse leukemia a
virus has been definitely isolated. This virus can cause leukemia
in mice. It can infect normal mouse cells, turning them into
malignant forms. Mice have been immunized against this virus.
If, then, a viral agent can be isolated from human cancer cells,
grown in pure culture and shown to reproduce the disease in
tissue culture, then immunization against certain types of cancer
becomes a distinct possibility.

Meanwhile, in the absence of an effective vaccine, and until the
time when the air can be cleared of carcinogens, cancer will be
with us, to be treated by the best available procedures of surgery,
radiation, and hopefully with an increasing array of new and
more effective chemical agents.

NOTE ON CONTRIBUTOR

Morris E. Friedkin (Ph.D., Biochemistry, 1948) is professor and chairman of the Department of Biochemistry at Tufts University School of Medicine. He holds a Ph.D. in biochemistry and was a postdoctoral fellow of the National Institutes of Health at the University of Copenhagen. He presently serves as consultant to the National Cancer Institute. Author of numerous articles in medical, biology, and chemistry journals, his research focus largely has been new concepts of biochemical action relating to cell growth mechanisms, particularly in relation to emergence or inhibition of malignant changes.

8

Drugs in the Prevention of Heart Attacks and Strokes

SAMUEL PROGER, M.D.

HEART ATTACKS AND STROKES together are the commonest causes of death in the United States. This problem was brought into sharp focus a few years ago by the President's commission on heart disease, cancer, and stroke, which pointed out that heart disease and stroke alone accounted for just over one-half (50.1 per cent) of all deaths in our country in 1963. To be sure, these deaths were predominantly in older people. But younger people also succumb to heart disease and strokes, especially heart disease. In fact, in 1963 this affliction killed a quarter of a million people in their most productive years, that is between the ages of 25 and 64. The President's commission found it worthwhile to note that had all in this young group lived just one more year, the economy would have gained some two billion dollars worth of output. But the commission was also keenly aware that statistics do not measure the heartbreak and long emotional stress that follow a parent's death. Nor do they express the personal economic hardship that comes in the wake of a father's sudden, fatal heart attack.

But even greater than the loss resulting from death is the loss through illness and disability from heart disease. It is estimated that nearly one-fourth of the adults among us already have, or run the risk of having heart disease in some form. This is a remarkable figure. Though it may provide a measure of the number of hours of idleness enforced by chronic disability, it does not, however, "measure the length of each hour." I do not need to belabor the fact that cardiovascular disease is clearly the greatest medical problem facing America today.

At best, the problem can only be lessened by treating the strokes and heart attacks after they occur. It will be eliminated or sharply reduced only through preventive measures. It is in this approach, namely prevention, that drugs will have their greatest opportunity to promote health and prolong life.

Thus far drugs have done very little to prevent deaths from heart attacks and strokes. Consequently, they have done very little to prolong life beyond middle age. The Metropolitan Life Insurance Company in its Statistical Bulletin noted that the expectation of life for white men at age sixty-five increased from 11.5 years in the period between 1900 and 1902 to 12.8 years in 1950. This increase of 1.3 years reflected largely the significant advances in public health measures and drug remedies as well as marked improvement in nutrition and living standards. These advances resulted in greatly reduced mortality from such illnesses as tuberculosis, pneumonia, and other infectious diseases. But in the period between 1950 and 1962 the life expectancy for white men at age sixty-five increased only from 12.8 years to 12.9 years, or practically none at all. Indications are that future gains in longevity will depend for the most part on advances against degenerative diseases; and the principal degenerative disease is atherosclerosis (often called arteriosclerosis) or hardening of the arteries. Hardening of the arteries leads to heart attacks or strokes, depending upon whether the arterial narrowing or closure involves the heart or the brain.

Atherosclerosis is to some extent a reflection of wear and tear on the inner lining of arteries and hence is probably not wholly preventable. However, if the atherosclerotic or hardening process cannot be prevented, there are reasons to believe that it can be slowed, and the subsequent appearance of heart attacks and strokes thereby delayed. The two chief reasons for such a belief are, first, that experimentally induced lesions in animals, somewhat analogous to those seen in human atherosclerosis, are preventable; and second, that some of the conditions in man thought to be responsible for accelerating the atherosclerotic process are correctable.

We have better data on heart attacks than on strokes. But atherosclerosis is the underlying problem in both conditions. So what I shall have to say about heart attacks applies in the main to strokes as well, at least those strokes that are due to a clot blocking an artery to the brain. This is the mechanism in some 75–80 per cent of all strokes. The remainder are due to a ruptured brain vessel.

THE PERSON PRONE TO CORONARY DISEASE

Certain people are more likely to have early heart attacks than others. We know how to identify with fair reliability those who are prone to early heart attacks and those who are not. For purposes of this discussion I shall separate the factors that identify the candidates for coronary attacks into two categories. There are the factors of inner origin, which are inherent in a person's makeup, and those of outer origin. The factors of inner origin (endogenous) are age, sex, diabetes, high blood fats (including cholesterol), and high blood pressure. The factors of outer origin (or exogenous) are poor dietary habits, lack of exercise, nervous tension, and cigarette smoking.

I have not included in the endogenous category factors such as obesity, heredity, personality characteristics, and body build. These are, to be sure, important factors but they appear to be important principally because of their relationship to three of the endogenous factors already mentioned; namely, high blood pressure, diabetes, and high blood fats. Thus heredity is important if one inherits a tendency to high blood pressure, high blood fats, or diabetes. It may not be very important otherwise so far as athero-sclerosis is concerned. The same may be said of obesity. There is a much higher incidence of diabetes and hypertension in fat people. As a result there is a higher incidence of heart attacks. If, on the other hand, the fat person has normal blood sugar, normal blood pressure, and normal blood fats, he may be no more likely to have a heart attack than his counterpart of normal weight. This is not to say that such a person should not lose weight. There are other health hazards associated with obesity which shorten life. Obesity is a highly undesirable state for many reasons.

The exogenous and endogenous factors to some extent are probably interrelated. Eating excessively may lead to obesity and obesity to diabetes. Eating improperly may raise the blood fats. Nervous tension may increase the blood pressure. Smoking ciga-rettes may raise the blood fats and elevate the blood pressure.

The exogenous factors are controllable. Indolence, gluttony, nervous tension, and cigarette smoking are not wholly unman-ageable. One can discipline one's self to exercise regularly and moderately, to eat properly, and to stop smoking. And one can even learn to respond more calmly to life's tensions. The endogenous factors present a different picture. One can do noth-ing about one's age or sex. The arterial damage that occurs in patients with diabetes may progress whether or not the diabetes is brought under control. With respect to the endogenous factors, one is left with the management of high blood pressure and high blood fats as the chief therapeutic measures for possibly slowing the atherosclerotic process.

THE RELATION OF HIGH BLOOD PRESSURE AND HIGH BLOOD FATS TO HEART ATTACKS

Heart attacks may and do occur at all levels of cholesterol and blood pressure. Blood pressure and blood fats are related to heart attacks in a linear fashion. That is to say, the higher the cholesterol or the higher the pressure, the greater the likelihood of a heart attack. The lower the pressure or the lower the cholesterol, the smaller the risk of a heart attack. There is no level below which there is no relation to heart attacks. This relationship is illustrated in the following charts containing data from the studies of the United States Public Health Service in Framingham.

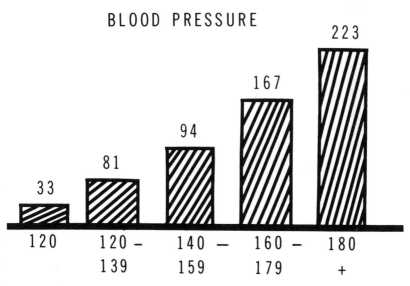

BLOOD PRESSURE

120	120 – 139	140 – 159	160 – 179	180 +
33	81	94	167	223

A man whose blood pressure at systole is higher than 160 runs five times the risk of heart attack than a man with systolic pressure under 120 runs (average heart attack rate = 100).

We do not know exactly why elevated blood pressure and cholesterol accelerate the atherosclerotic process, although there are many theoretical reasons why they might do so. The damaging effect of high blood pressure on the vessel wall is probably due to purely mechanical factors; that is the pressure and flow of blood associated with turbulence and suction. The mechanical factors appear to produce areas of injury at predictably vulnerable sites. These favored areas for the development of atheroscle-

rotic lesions in the arteries are at their branchings, turns, narrow-
ings, and attachments. It is in such areas that the potentially
damaging hydrodynamic (more properly hemodynamic) effects
are most pronounced.

The atherosclerotic lesion on the inner lining of the arteries is

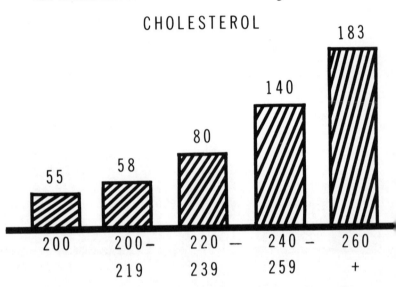

A man with a blood cholesterol measurement of 260 or more runs
more than three times the risk than one with cholesterol less than 200
runs (average heart attack rate = 100).

a raised, fatty, and fibrous area, called a placque. It represents, in
effect, the response of the arterial lining to injury either mechanical or inflammatory. The response will be either that of healing
or of degeneration. The fibrous portion is the healed scar, the
fatty portion is the degenerated tissue. The fatty, degenerative
process is probably related to the fat content of the blood that
bathes the vessel wall. Understandably the degeneration may be
expected to be more pronounced the higher the content of fat. It
is probably for this reason that high blood fats including cholesterol are associated with a higher incidence of heart attacks. It is

because of this association that attempts are made to lower blood cholesterol.

High blood fats can often be lowered moderately by diet. And high blood pressure can be lowered somewhat by minimizing stress, but this approach is obviously of limited value. It appears that we shall need more effective means for lowering blood pressure and blood fats if we are going to decrease significantly the death rate from heart attacks. We look to drugs to supply these means.

As I have already indicated, the evidence is convincing that high blood pressure and high blood fats are associated with more frequent and earlier heart attacks. It does not necessarily follow that lowering blood pressure and blood fats will delay or eliminate the heart attacks. The evidence, however, is sufficiently suggestive to justify the widespread use of drugs for this purpose, if the drugs are safe, easily administered, and not too costly. It is only in the past decade that we have had drugs that begin to meet these qualifications. In this period the history of the discovery of satisfactory drugs for the control of high blood pressure and the lowering of blood fats has been a history of the effective collaboration of university scientists, clinical investigators, and the pharmaceutical industry.

THE TREATMENT OF HIGH BLOOD PRESSURE

As I view it, the development of antihypertensive treatment seems to have proceeded along two separate lines. The first dealt with the relationship of salt to blood pressure. In the early 1920's it was first suggested that a low-salt diet was beneficial in patients with high blood pressure. However, the evidence for such benefit was not sufficiently convincing to persuade people of the merits of so tasteless a diet. Indeed, Sir George Pickering of Oxford, England, thought so poorly of a low-salt diet that he quoted the King in *Alice Through the Looking Glass,* who said, "There is nothing like eating hay when you're faint. . . . I didn't say there is nothing better, I just said there is nothing like it." So physicians heard little more about the relation of salt restriction to blood pressure until Walter Kempner, at Duke University, introduced the so-called rice diet in the 1940's. From the gourmet's point of view rice might have been little better than hay, but there was considerable enthusiasm for it. As Irvine H. Page of Cleveland said of the rice diet, it "had a certain aura and allure to it. It was recommended with almost religious fervor. You had to start by believing! . . . But unsalted rice and fruit juice was a form of medical mayhem. . . ." More and more it came to be the feeling, as Page put it, that the Chinese could have it. It was a research team in Dallas that showed what the rice diet's real virtue was in hypertension: It was its extremely low salt content. The salt that I refer to is ordinary table salt, namely sodium chloride, of which the sodium is the important element. The diet is more properly, therefore, a low sodium diet. But the severe dietary restriction of salt, to the degree it was comparable to that of the rice diet, proved impractical; especially since it appeared that salt restriction had to be continued for a lifetime. There was reason to believe that the same effect might be obtained by the use of drugs that would effectively deplete the body of sodium, or at least drastically reduce the amount of sodium retained in the tissues. The idea was to increase the sodium eliminated in the urine instead of decreasing the sodium in food or drink. The first of such drugs, called diuretics, used to treat high blood pressure, was developed in the laboratories of the drug manufacturers, Merck, Sharp and Dohme. This drug, known as chlorothiazide, proved very effective in lowering high blood pressure. It was a key factor in advancing the treatment of hypertension.

Incidentally, it is still not clear why the elimination of sodium helps lower blood pressure, or if indeed it is the loss of sodium that is responsible. As so often happens in medicine, remedies are found first and the reasons for their effectiveness are then slowly, if ever, discovered.

The story of the second major approach to the treatment of

high blood pressure is also interesting. In this, the idea was to modify the effects that the nervous system has on the diameter or caliber of the arteries. The walls of blood vessels are composed in part of smooth muscle. If they are under tension, the vessel is narrow, and the pressure in it is correspondingly high. If the wall muscle is somehow persuaded to relax, the vessel widens and the pressure falls.

The caliber of the arteries is regulated by the sympathetic nervous system. Through it stimuli are constantly being sent to the smooth muscle of the arteries to maintain a degree of muscular tension in the arterial wall. The problem then was to block this sympathetic nerve stimulus.

The first approach to this, also in the 1920's, was direct. Adson, a neurosurgeon at the Mayo Clinic in Minnesota, simply cut the sympathetic nerves of the abdomen where they emerged from the lumbar spine. The technique went by the name *lumbar sympathectomy*. This operation proved ineffective. Shortly thereafter the sympathetic nerves in the chest were cut (*dorsal or thoracic sympathectomy*—a technique developed by Max Peet at the University of Michigan). This operation was occasionally successful. Perhaps somewhat more success was achieved by cutting both the lumbar and dorsal nerves (*lumbo-dorsal sympathectomy*). This was the operation made famous by Reginald Smithwick in Boston. But surgical sympathectomy was an extremely radical approach that could be justified only in the most serious cases; and most patients with high blood pressure do not have the serious form of the disease. There had to be a simpler approach. Hence, the attempt to block sympathetic nerve stimulation by drugs. Here again the contributions of the drug industry, working in close collaboration with laboratory and clinical investigators in universities and research institutes, have been outstanding. There are now drugs that block the constricting effect of the nerves on arteries, and other drugs that facilitate the removal of salt. There are still others that lower blood pressure through still different mechanisms.

In medicine the judicious combination of various therapies is often more effective than the use of any one of them. This is true in the treatment of hypertension, and the combined use of two or more methods of controlling high blood pressure usually results in truly effective treatment.

Now that we have the means for controlling high blood pressure, the central questions remain: What effect will the widespread control of hypertension have on the atherosclerotic process? Will it slow the hardening of the arteries and thereby prolong productive life? We shall soon know, and there is reason to believe that the answer will be favorable.

Circumstances surrounding the treatment of high bood pressure provide a classic example of a common therapeutic dilemma; that is, under what conditions can we justify the use of drugs that are only presumably helpful? Many drugs fall into this category. Before embarking on the use of such drugs, one must ask a number of questions. Concerning the drug, one must ask, for example: Has it been adequately tested; how difficult is it to administer; is there full knowledge of the possible early and late side effects, their recognition and control; how costly is it? With respect to the illness one must query: How serious is it; if it is not serious, how troublesome is it; how likely is it to subside spontaneously; how helpful would simple reassurance be, or some inert substance like a placebo? At times, when balancing such sets of questions, the answer is obvious. This was the case with respect to some of the early attempts to treat hypertension, medical as well as surgical. It was then clear that mild to moderate elevations of blood pressure were less hazardous than the treatments then in vogue. The same could be said of the drug treatment of high blood fats. One illustration is the ill-fated experience with MER-29, a drug widely used just a few years ago. But circumstances have now changed with respect to the drug treatment of high blood pressure and high blood fats. The factors that determine the ratio of drug efficacy to drug safety are at present such as to favor drugs. Indeed, the general view now is that conditions favoring drug treatment justify their widespread use in most patients with at least moderately severe hypertension and certainly in patients with severe hypertension. We are approaching the same position with respect to the drug treatment of high blood cholesterol.

Our experience with these drugs illustrates another point of great importance in the use of new drugs. I refer to the difficulty, or at least the delay, that often occurs in recognizing harmful side effects. Chlorothiazide is an example. This diuretic eliminates sodium, to be sure, but physicians immediately noted that it also caused loss of sodium's sister element, potassium. Depletion of the body's potassium is always undesirable and sometimes can produce damaging effects, especially on the kidneys. The answer was to give potassium supplements to the patient along with the diuretic.

A more serious side effect of the thiazides was not observable for many months after the diuretics went into general use. Then physicians noticed that gout and diabetes were appearing in patients who had been free of either disease. In fact even the drugs used to prevent complications may themselves cause difficulties. Hence the potassium supplements given in enteric-coated tablets, for the purpose of replacing the potassium loss, were found, many months later, to cause occasional intestinal ulceration and obstruction.

The moral of the tale is that the long-term use of any new drug may produce late, and unexpected, harmful effects. Before a physician can be entirely certain that a drug is doing more good than harm, he must cautiously observe for years the effects of a drug. We now have sufficient experience with antihypertensive drugs to be satisfied that, if they are properly used, their benefits outweigh the occasional complications. But note the qualifying phrase, "if properly used." This is a most important aspect of the use of any new drug. When a new drug is introduced and appears promising, there is a tendency for it to be widely and uncritically prescribed. Some of this improper use is the result of the natural enthusiasm of both patients and physicians for something new. And some of it is the result of understandable but unfortunately excessive promotion by the drug industry. How else can we account for the prescribing of 600 million thiazide tablets in 1961 or for 7.4 million *new* prescriptions—each for more than a single tablet, of course—for diuretics or combinations of them in 1964? But the excessive and uncritical use of a drug should not cause it to be abandoned, any more than its benefits should encourage its indiscriminate distribution.

THE TREATMENT OF HIGH BLOOD CHOLESTEROL

So much for the drug treatment of high blood pressure. We come now to the treatment of high blood cholesterol. As I have indicated, certain dietary measures will occasionally result in a modest lowering of blood cholesterol. At present these dietary measures involve chiefly a decreased intake of animal fats (saturated fats) with supplements of vegetable oils (unsaturated fats). There remains, nonetheless, an important place for drugs. Many drugs are said to lower blood cholesterol. A recent monograph on atherosclerosis lists forty-nine of them; but only a few have been used to any extent in recent years in this country. These are female hormones, thyroid preparations, and nicotinic acid. All have disturbing disadvantages. The female hormones, if given to males in doses sufficient to alter the blood fats, have a feminizing effect, notably an enlargement of the breasts. Thyroid preparations, while they lower blood cholesterol, also often induce angina pectoris, or aggravate pre-existing angina pectoris. And nicotinic acid, which must be given indefinitely in order to maintain its effect on blood fats, may have immediate troublesome and delayed serious side-effects. The delayed effects include the development of diabetes, gout, or disturbed liver function. With one exception, there are important limitations to the use of all the drugs that have been found to lower blood fats. The one exception is a drug developed by the Imperial Chemical Industries of England and known by the trade name Atromid-S.

The history of the development of Atromid-S is of interest. This history begins with the observation already mentioned that thyroid hormone lowers blood cholesterol. But this hormone increases the work of the heart. And as I have pointed out, it may induce angina pectoris. The ideal thyroid preparation would be one that had only the cholesterol lowering effect; but no such preparation could be developed. It was noted, however, that patients who have overactive thyroid glands and hence low blood cholesterol, have an increased amount of a substance in the urine that derives from the breakdown of a masculinizing hormone in the adrenal gland. This substance is called androsterone. Could androsterone have anything to do with the fat-lowering effect of the thyroid hormone? When tested in animals, androsterone was indeed found to lower the blood cholesterol. But androsterone was impractical as a therapeutic agent. When given by mouth, even in high doses and despite adequate absorption, it was active for only minutes. It was at this point that research chemists in the British chemical firm entered the picture. They found that by combining small amounts of androsterone with a special salt, a combination that could be taken by mouth, the desired lowering of the blood cholesterol could be achieved and maintained. This salt is quite unlike sodium chloride or table salt. It goes by the forbidding name of ethyl chlorophenoxyisobutyrate. The salt alone subsequently proved to be as effective as the combination with androsterone, so that it is now given without the androsterone. It has been widely tested in animals and in human beings, is effective, and after a considerable experience of more than five years, seems to be relatively free of undesirable side effects. Just how it produces its effects is not known.

It appears that we now have a safe and efficacious drug that will lower blood cholesterol. We may soon expect, therefore, to have conclusive information as to whether lowering the blood cholesterol will retard the atherosclerotic process and thus eliminate or delay the appearance of heart attacks and strokes.

THE PREVENTION OF ARTERIAL CLOTS

In the prevention of heart attacks and strokes we are concerned not alone with lowering blood pressure and blood fats. We should like also to be able to prevent the plugging of an artery in the heart or brain by a clot, or more properly a thrombus. Such a closure of an artery in the heart is called coronary thrombosis; in the brain, cerebral thrombosis. For many years, anticlotting drugs, called *anticoagulants,* have been used in the hope that they would decrease the likelihood of a thrombus forming in and blocking a blood vessel. Generally speaking, the anticlotting drugs have not been as effective as we had hoped. All physicians are not equally impressed with their benefits in preventing heart attacks and strokes. Indeed, there are some who believe them to be of no value.

The experience with anticoagulants typifies some of the difficult problems encountered in evaluating drugs. It is some twenty years since anticoagulants have been recommended and extensively used in the treatment of heart attacks, that is in the acute episodes. Yet there is a persistent disagreement as to their benefits, and the choice of patients to whom they should be administered. If such a lack of agreement exists in the treatment of a disease that requires controlled studies for only a few weeks, it is not surprising that there is even greater controversy regarding the benefits of long-term anticlotting treatment in preventing heart attacks and strokes. It requires a study of many people over a period of years to answer the question of whether heart attacks and strokes are in fact prevented.

However, the over-all evidence appears to justify, in some patients, long-term anticoagulant treatment for the prevention of heart attacks. The benefits seem more definite during the first year of treatment after an attack, and especially in males under fifty-five years of age. The treatment requires careful supervision by the physician and periodic examinations of the blood to check the level of anticlotting effect.

OTHER POSSIBLY HELPFUL MEASURES

If heart attacks and strokes cannot be entirely prevented, we should like to be able to minimize their effects when they do occur. For this purpose, measures are aimed at stimulating the development of new vessels or "stand-by vessels" that can take over some of the flow of blood when an artery is blocked. Obviously this needs to be done in advance. With effective new vessel formation the extent of a stroke may be lessened and the size of a heart attack decreased. In this area drugs seem to be of limited value.

CIGARETTE SMOKING

Earlier I referred to cigarette smoking as an exogenous factor in the incidence of heart attacks and strokes. A discussion of this subject is appropriate here because tobacco contains a drug, nicotine, the elimination of which might prevent or postpone heart attacks and strokes.

The nicotine effect of cigarette smoking is clear and demonstrable. Nicotine results in a quickening of the heart rate, an elevation of blood pressure, and a release of fatty acids from body depots of fat. Again we find the factors of increased blood pressure and blood fats coming into play. But whether or not these factors are responsible, the fact is that cigarette smoking (one pack or more a day) is regularly associated with increased deaths from heart attacks. In this regard the studies undertaken by the United States Public Health Service in Albany, New York, and in Framingham, Massachusetts, are impressive. In these two cities the smoking habits of 4,120 men were studied. At the beginning of the study there were 1,838 men, thirty-nine to fifty-five years old, residing in Albany and 2,282 men, thirty to sixty-two years old, residing in Framingham. The Albany group had been observed for six years and the Framingham group for eight years when the joint report was published in 1962. The significant findings—and they appear highly significant—were first, that heavy cigarette smokers had almost three times as many heart attacks (myocardial infarctions) as nonsmokers; and second, and even more important, in those who had stopped smoking, morbidity and mortality statistics were similar to those who had never smoked. Cigar and pipe smokers had the same favorable experience as nonsmokers. Additional observations of these groups of subjects since the report in 1962 have confirmed the original findings, as have similar studies by others. These are noteworthy figures. Especially impressive, as I have indicated, is the observation that almost immediately after stopping cigarette smoking, illness and mortality from heart attacks declines to that of nonsmokers. I have previously pointed out that while high blood pressure and high blood fats are known to be associated with a higher death rate from heart attacks, we do not yet have proof that lowering the blood pressure and blood fats will lower the death rate. With respect to the factor of cigarette smoking, however, there is evidence that its removal will eliminate the excess of the associated heart deaths. When we realize that up to two-thirds of all heart deaths due to coronary disease in cigarette smokers may be prevented by the simple expedient of stopping cigarette smoking, we begin to comprehend the magnitude of the preventive possibilities. There is probably no area in medicine today in which preventive measures have more to offer.

The approach to the problem of cigarette smoking is basically one of public health education. A program of public health education, to be successful, must counter the extremely effective advertising programs of the cigarette companies. These advertising programs seem to be directed toward a single goal, that of somehow equating cigarette smoking with the good life. On the other hand, the aim of public health officials and practicing physicians has been to equate stopping of cigarette smoking with a long life. The issue comes down to an apparent choice between the good life and the long life, and the vote has gone overwhelmingly, especially among young people, in favor of the good cigarette-smoking life. It has been an unequal contest and a false one, because the public needs to be shown that one can have both a long life and a good one without cigarettes.

I have discussed those risk factors with respect to heart attacks

CIGARETTE SMOKING

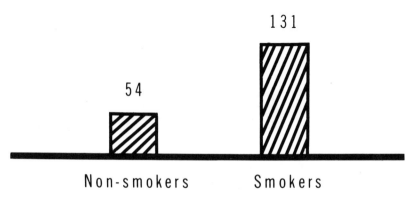

A man who smokes one pack or more of cigarettes a day runs more than twice the risk of a non-smoker (average heart attack rate = 100).

and strokes that bear some relation to drugs. These are high blood pressure, high blood fats, and cigarette smoking. Each factor is significant. In combination they assume even more significance.

The importance of eliminating these risk factors in the prevention of heart attacks and strokes would appear to be self-evident.

THE FUTURE

There is reason to anticipate that the medical profession will make progress in its efforts to reduce heart attacks and strokes, or at least delay their appearance. To prevent heart attacks and strokes is to prolong life. The prolongation of life will inevitably create social and economic problems not unrelated to those of uncontrolled birth rates. The social and economic problems will

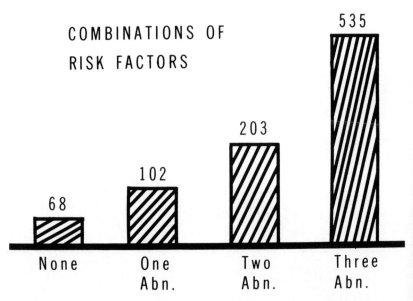

Combinations of two or more factors compound the risk of a heart attack. Abnormalities: cholesterol, 250 or more; blood pressure, 160 or more; smoking, more than one pack of cigarettes per day (average heart attack rate = 100).

not just be those of an increased population but of an increased older population. It is none too early to begin to plan for this eventuality.

More older people without less younger people will obviously compound the problem of unmanageable population growth. In prolonging life we shall have to curtail births. If we have more old people, we shall have to have fewer new people. We should then be left with a population with an average age higher than that of our present population (it was 28.5 years in 1963). If the

older people remain mentally alert and physically fit, we shall find ourselves with a more experienced, a more mature, and perhaps a wiser and more reasonable society. Such an older society might approach world problems somewhat differently from our present society. Whether this would result in more or less progress, and in what direction, is hard to predict. There are those who believe a change could hardly be for the worse.

I believe that we need not fear the effects of an increased older population if this means that more people will have a longer period of health and usefulness. Health and usefulness are companions to happiness and productivity. And to have more happy and productive people is, after all, among the highest of human aims. This then, in effect, is the ultimate purpose of drugs in the prevention of heart attacks and strokes.

NOTE ON CONTRIBUTOR

Samuel Proger (M.D., 1928, Emory University, Atlanta, Georgia) is physician-in-chief of the New England Medical Center Hospitals and Louisa C. Endicott Professor and chairman of the Department of Medicine, Tufts University School of Medicine, Boston, Massachusetts. He is also president of the Bingham Associates Fund for the Advancement of Medicine. His major research interests are diseases of the heart and blood vessels, a field to which he has made many clinical and physiological contributions. A member of several national medical, cardiovascular, and research societies, he has also served on the executive committee of the scientific council of the American Heart Association; as president of the Massachusetts Heart Association and New England Cardiovascular Society.

9

Diseases Due to Drug Treatment

COLONEL ROBERT H. MOSER,
MC, U.S. ARMY

THE CONTEMPORARY PHYSICAN and his patient are benefi-
ciaries of the most dramatic expansion of capability in the
long history of our art. But the rapid proliferation of medical
knowledge has not been entirely benign. Our reverses have been
minor when contrasted to our advances, but negative effects
cannot be ignored or derogated. This presentation is concerned
with one aspect of this problem—the emergence of what I have
chosen to call "Diseases of Medical Progress." These could be
paraphrased as "diseases-that-would-not-have-occurred-if-sound-
medical-treatment-had-not-been-employed." Despite the offen-
sive double negative, what I mean is "diseases caused by drugs"
—usually given for good reason.

Improvement in quantity and quality of drugs is, of course,
pertinent to the evolution of medical capability. But in the early
days of this century new drugs came in a trickle: There was time
for the physician to become familiar with their virtues and idio-
syncrasies. Soon, however, the trickle became a stream. There
was less time for study and reflection. The stream has now be-

come a torrent; and it is impossible for the physician to keep pace. His little black bag runneth over.

It has been said that adverse patient reactions induced by drugs is the price we pay for more effective and better medicaments. There can be no quarrel with this statement. It is the high price we are haggling about. The thalidomide disaster indicated how expensive it can be.

The deluge of new drugs has created a widespread spirit of discontent with empiricism in therapeutics. The modern practitioner demands drugs that have proper credentials, and this has precipitated a virtual renaissance in drug investigation. Thus we have come to learn more of the wonders—and hazards—of contemporary therapeutic agents.

Present-day demands of the clinician to know more about drugs are being met by increased capability in the laboratory. New insight and appreciation of the complexities of drug effects have come from several diverse avenues of investigation. We now have simple methods for obtaining tissue specimens from many organs. And we enjoy improved techniques for examining such tissues. The all-seeing electron microscope and more sophisticated methods of preparing the tissue have resulted in dramatic revelations. The mysteries of life within individual cells in the living organism have begun to yield. Often we are able to observe the specific site of action of a given drug within the cell and even, at times, within subcellular structures.

In other areas techniques continue to be perfected for measurement of blood and tissue levels of drugs, their intermediate degradation products and enzymes. But the problems of adverse drug effects are many.

Reduced to its simplest terms, when Drug A is introduced into the body, ultimately it will be carried in blood and other body fluids to almost all cells of the human organism. The effects of Drug A become perceptible only when the function of certain organs is modified to the point of producing obvious changes. These may be beneficial or harmful. For example, if the organ is

the failing heart, and Drug *A* is digitalis, we will recognize its presence by improvement in function of the heart. Of course this is beneficial. However, if the organ is the liver and Drug *A* happens to be, let us say, the male hormone methyltestosterone, the patient may become jaundiced, and this would be harmful. Thus it is by these phenomena that we learn to characterize the nature of Drug *A*. As we focus our attention upon the response of a specific organ or organs to this drug, however, we are inclined to forget that Drug *A* is also bathing other tissues. Effects in these nontarget areas are not in immediate evidence, but subtle changes may be taking place, which may not cause untoward or fortuitous signs or symptoms until a much later date. Long-range effects may never be correlated with the antecedent administration of our Drug *A*.

Only painstaking retrospective analysis of many cases will reveal that in all probability it was our friend Drug *A* that was the benefactor or malefactor, as the case may be. Then we must set about proving it. We must design a prospective study which will involve clinical testing. That is, we must administer Drug *A* under carefully controlled circumstances to appropriate animals before we can prove, for example, that indeed it was Drug *A* that caused a chronic disease. Such provocative testing in human subjects is, of course, often not feasible.

This is a shadow world involving the interaction of drugs and tissues where relation of cause-to-effect is, at best, very difficult to assess. I need only cite the heated dialogue between physicians that still persists over the pain-killing analgesic agent, phenacetin, and its possible contribution to kidney disease, to demonstrate the difficulty.

An example of the effect of drugs in accelerating degenerative disease would be the influence of prolonged administration of cortisone, and its synthetic cousins, in the elderly patient immobilized by heart disease or arthritis. In this situation the drug, via an interference with normal tissue formation, may cause a rapid leaching of calcium and protein from bones. We start with one disease, and our treatment for it—based upon sound judgment and given with hope and good intention—produces another disease.

Let us modify the question again. What is known of the effects of drugs upon a previously diseased organ, particularly one with limited capacity to detoxify or otherwise cope with the drug given to treat another illness? In this regard the phenacetin controversy again serves to illustrate the issue. This discussion revolves around the possible role of certain pain-relieving drugs in provoking an infection in a normal kidney. But what effect does phenacetin or aspirin have on the sick kidney, already poorly disposed to resist assault from either bacteria or drugs known to be occasionally toxic to kidneys?

Consider for a moment, too, the patient with inapparent liver disease. Let us say he has had slowly progressive scarring of his liver over the course of years, but without developing overt signs or symptoms. Let us suppose he becomes nervous, and is given chlorpromazine, a tranquilizer known to be occasionally toxic to the liver. How does this already damaged organ manage to cope under such circumstances? And there are perhaps fifty drugs that could be considered in this context.

One could cite many other examples wherein an organ with marginal function may be further insulted by a drug administered to treat another ailing system.

Perhaps the most fascinating corollary to these observations is the identification of a relationship between enzyme systems and drug effects. In 1959 Dr. F. Vogel of West Germany introduced the term "pharmacogenetics" into clinical medicine. He defined the term as "the study of genetically determined variations that are revealed solely by the effects of drugs." Genetic variation results in the absence or insufficiency of certain enzyme systems required to detoxify certain drugs. This mechanism has already been cited as one major explanation of the frequently encountered, individual variation-and-response to conventional doses of conventional drugs. Brevity precludes a discussion here of these intriguing and complex disorders, but there are easily a dozen known congenital enzyme insufficiencies already identified. In view of the multitude of known enzyme systems, as well as those suspected but not as yet identified, one could predict that many adverse drug reactions, now attributed to idiosyncrasy or hypersensitivity of individuals, will soon be classified as pharmacogenetic disorders or the results of acquired enzyme insufficiencies.

A related phenomenon is the inhibition of the breakdown of one drug by yet another. For example, Drug *A* is given along with Drug *B*. Drug *B* then interferes with the breakdown of Drug *A*. Thus, Drug *A* will persist in the blood or tissues for a longer time than normally is the case. An illustration of this is the potentiation of the effects of anticlotting drugs, the anticoagulants often used in the management of occlusive blood vessel disease. This potentiation-of-effect may be caused by a series of drugs, including aspirin, phenylbutazone, and some common antibiotics. Thus, in this situation, the dosage of the anticoagulant would have to be lowered, or given less frequently.

Now we also have a new dimension, quite antithetical to the concepts of congenital enzyme deficiencies or the inhibition of one drug by another. I refer to the phenomenon called "enzyme induction" in which the administration of one drug actually accelerates the metabolic breakdown of another. Here, Drug *A* is given, and when Drug *B* is administered, it greatly accelerates the breakdown of Drug *A*. Thus Drug *A* will have to be given more frequently or in higher dosage than normally. This can be seen where anticoagulants are given in conjunction with barbiturates. Often the dosage of anticoagulants must be increased if they are to be effective.

Residual drug effects are another enigma. For example, the anti-high blood pressure agent, reserpine, continues to exert its influence in certain patients for several weeks after it has been discontinued. Among its effects may be unpredictable responses to general anesthesia. There are many other known instances of residual effects. Agents may lie dormant for weeks to years, apparently innocuous, in curious contradiction to the usual tendency of the body to rid itself of foreign substances. It may be vital to know what other drugs are stored for prolonged periods. Do they exert adverse effects? The questions come easily; but the answers do not.

And finally, an equally fascinating new aspect of drug mechanisms is revealed in the recently recognized phenomenon of hereditary transference of drug resistance from one generation of bacteria to the next. This was first observed in Japan in 1959 during studies on the bacteria, shigella, a cause of dysentery. Shigella was then discovered to be resistant to several antibiotics, to which it formerly had been sensitive. It was subsequently recognized that both the bacteria, shigella, and also salmonella—both colon organisms—are capable of genetic transmission of drug resistance. It has been suggested that the widespead use of antibacterial agents in agricultural feeds has contributed to this problem. To my knowledge, genetically transferred resistance factors have been identified only in certain specific bacterial species.

Now that you have survived this dry recitation describing some of the mischief that can be set in motion when you swallow that pill, I will strain your tolerance just a bit more. A logical question might be: What will be the ultimate outcome of these new therapeutic endeavors? The answer must lie somewhat in the misty interface between philosophy and physiology.

The evolution of man is a continuing source of wonderment to students of physiology. Through centuries of painful metamorphosis, each challenge thrown at man by his environment was met by gradual genetic adaptation that enabled man to survive. The species has arrived at the current state of advanced physiological capability, a state admirably suited to its environment. We can dig diamonds 9,000 feet underground in 123° heat and 100 per cent humidity; we can spend a lifetime mining tin at 14,900 feet elevation; we can hike across the polar regions of the earth; and we can float—weightless—in space for fourteen days.

But in the past few decades we have devised methods to challenge the adaptability of the organism that are unprecedented in the entire previous experience of the species. We have designed molecules unique to human physiology and have intruded them into blood and tissue by techniques that are also unique in physiologic experience. Intravenous, intramuscular, and subcutaneous injections, positive pressure inhalation, rectal administration, and even passage through intact skin; all are unfamiliar modes of gaining access to the body. Add radiation—by X-ray, beta ray, gamma ray, and neutrons—plus oxygen under greatly increased barometric pressure and some other modes of application that I have doubtless forgotten, and you begin to appreciate the magnitude and genius of man's conspiracy to by-pass the conventional avenues for introducing new environmental factors to the physiology of man.

In the past we had to cope only with naïve nature and unsubtle environment. And they were restricted to the gastrointestinal tract, the lungs, and occasionally the abraded skin as available avenues for admission of alien materials to the core of man.

The implications of these ingenious new tactics of assault, these strange man-made chemicals and emanations upon the beleaguered human mechanism, are fascinating to contemplate. One could philosophize that this incredibly resilient physiological machine of ours is sufficiently advanced in design to be able to cope with all transgressors. We have evolved defenses at all levels from the simplest neurologic reflex to the most complex immune reactions to meet the daily challenges of environment. And we have done very well in the matter of self-preservation.

Yet it is a fact of medical history that some of these unprecedented therapeutic intrusions overtax the ability of the body to accommodate, and it reacts with displeasure if not violent rejection. This is, of course, close to the heart of our thesis—drug-induced diseases.

And now that I have indulged in this reverie all the way into shade-tree philosophy, I will proceed to specifics. Every new drug must be evaluated for efficacy and toxicity, and this is not an easy task. Only passage of time and acquisition of experience will determine the ultimate verdict. Firm pronouncements based on animal experimentation or fragmentary early clinical trials are premature and meaningless. Often it takes years before the full spectrum of efficacy or toxicity of a drug becomes evident. This poses an almost insoluble conundrum. If we are timid and withhold the drug, how will we ever gain the necessary clinical experience? If the agent is effective and safe, it would seem unfair to hold it back. But, alternatively, if the drug is ineffective or unduly toxic, it would seem equally unjust to use it on patients. All that one can propose is prudence, caution, and reservation of final judgment until objective studies are completed.

I would enjoy taking you on a panoramic trip through the fascinating landscape of drug-induced diseases; an area which has occupied my interest for the past decade. But this would make my narrative too lengthy. Consequently, in an effort to dramatize the problem of drug toxicity, I have selected one group of drugs, the adrenal cortical hormones, cortisone or corticosteroids. They will serve as prototypes, illustrating the continuing challenge that faces the medical profession in arriving at a comprehensive appreciation of the spectrum of toxic effects of drugs. One might select almost any popular drug and do the same thing. This discussion could properly be called the evolution of the toxic profile of a useful drug.

Corticosteroids are valuable therapeutic allies. They qualify as drugs of choice in a host of diseases. So let it be established at the outset that there is no denying the efficacy of corticosteroids in clinical medicine.

Perhaps no other drug can present a more dramatic and well-documented claim to the appellation *wonder drug* than the adrenal cortical hormones—the corticosteroids, epitomized by cortisone, hydrocortisone, and their myriad of synthetic cousins. The introduction of cortisone into clinical medicine was attended by fanfare rivaled only by penicillin and poliomyelitis vaccine.

Newspapers carried wild tales of hospital corridor histrionics with patients, long-crippled with rheumatoid arthritis, dancing in the corridors. The characteristic flurry of initial, uncritical, over-enthusiastic, uncontrolled reports caused an ominous ripple throughout the medical community. Cortisone is a hormone critical to normal physiologic function. Definite diseases are related to its underproduction (Addison's Disease) and overproduction (Cushing's Disease). However, the contagious rapture of early reports of the drug's efficacy in rheumatoid arthritis spilled over into other areas. Soon cortisone was being used in a wide assortment of disorders. The principal indication for the corticosteroids' employment seemed to be that no pre-existing mode of treatment had been effective. Near miraculous results were observed in such incredibly diverse conditions as pemphigus vulgaris—a fatal skin disorder; thrombocytopenic purpura—a bleeding disease caused by strange disappearance of blood-borne platelets (cells essential for clotting); nephrotic syndrome—a kidney disease characterized by massive urinary loss of serum albumin; as well as asthma, acute leukemia, thyroiditis, and acute hepatitis. And these were just a few.

With many drugs it takes years for significant adverse reactions to be observed. With these powerful agents, however, severe untoward effects were observed very quickly. Most were related to an exaggeration of the normal physiologic role of cortisone. (The familiar disease caused by overproduction of cortisone is called Cushing's Disease.) The use of cortisone in doses that were in excess of the body's normal physiologic production caused an identical series of events to those which occur in the disease. Rounding of the face, a peculiar obesity limited to hips and abdomen, acne, wasting of muscles of the extremities with attendant weakness, purple streaks due to stretching of the skin over the lateral portions of the abdomen and hips, and the growth of a peculiar soft tissue lump over the spine of the upper back—all of these were visible manifestations of prolonged high cortisone dosage.

A plethora of reports of peculiar psychological behavior ranging from euphoria (dancing in the corridors?) to profound depressions culminating in dramatic suicides were seen. The entire gamut of psychiatric disorders could be simulated in patients on cortisone therapy.

We also observed rises in blood pressure, possibly due to salt retention; a diabetes-like picture; and more subtle phenomena such as profound weakness due to urinary potassium loss. Cortisone also was known to exert profound metabolic changes, including a disturbance of normal production of tissue protein. This was manifested by a mysterious wasting of muscles, leaching of calcium and protein from bones with collapse of vertebral bodies, increased fragility of the fine capillary blood vessels with subcutaneous bleeding, and impaired healing of surgical wounds. All of these were observed in a significant proportion of patients receiving cortisone and cortisonelike drugs.

The ripple on the waters of this therapeutic paradise soon became a frightening wave. Editorials appeared in leading medical journals deploring the widespread indiscriminate use of the powerful drugs. Some authors became frankly panicked and advocated withdrawal of these drugs from clinical medicine. Such a backlash would have been more unfortunate than the lack of therapeutic prudence that had provoked it. The pendulum was oscillating with alarming rapidity, powered by an emotional heat unprecedented in the history of therapeutics.

But even at that point the full spectrum of adverse effects had not been revealed in all its florid glory.

In the course of corticosteroid treatment of patients with rheumatoid arthritis, a small percentage developed destruction of weight-bearing joint interfaces. This occurred insidiously; while the symptoms were improved, the X-rays indicated progressive deterioration. Further, on rare occasions the injection of cortisone congeners into joint spaces was attended by introduction of bacteria into the vulnerable joint fluid. Of course this is a hazard with all such injections, but the bacteria seemed to flourish in the corticosteroid-enriched environment. In addition the signs of inflammation that are the hallmarks of such an infection were often delayed due to the effect of the hormone.

This was a prelude to recognition of the strange liaison between corticosteroids and infections. These drugs possess the ability to suppress inflammatory reactions and mask the signs and symptoms of infection. In certain diseases the decrease in swelling (caused by exudation of fluid) is highly desirable, but the obfuscation of the danger signals of infection is a grave menace. The patient taking corticosteroids for asthma or rheumatoid arthritis or nephrotic syndrome could develop an acute appendicitis or pneumonia—without the attendant classical alerting signs and symptoms.

In an analogous area it was discovered that corticosteroids could facilitate the spread and propagation of an infection. Unless appropriate antibiotics were administered concomitantly, tuberculosis, blood stream bacterial infections, virus and fungus infections, would thrive under the stimulus of high dose corticosteroids given for another disease. To complicate the issue even further, it was later discovered that in certain overwhelming bacterial diseases the combination of corticosteroids and antibiotics could be lifesaving.

Among the earlier complications recognized as being attributable to corticosteroids was ulcer of the stomach. There was some conflicting evidence on this point, but the general consensus is that the association between corticosteroids and large ulcers of lesser curvature of the stomach is quite real.

The panorama of adverse reactions continued to expand: (1) A peculiar disorder characterized by joint discomfort in which fatigue, weakness, numbness, and mental depression occurred in some patients receiving corticosteroids with no change in dosage. (2) These drugs were noted to aggravate disease characterized by arterial damage (arteritis). (3) In some instances corticosteroids were observed to benefit a strange disease of the connective tissue called systemic lupus erythematosus; and paradoxically, in rare instances these drugs were thought to precipitate systemic lupus erythematosus in a patient who had never had it previously. (4) Cases of corticosteroid-induced inflammation of the pancreas (especially in children) were reported. (5) It was estimated that between 9 to 60 per cent of patients receiving high dose, long-term corticosteroid developed opacification of the lens portion of the eye with visual impairment in many. (6) Patients with one particular variety of glaucoma ("open angle") showed an increase in pressure within the eyeball while receiving corticosteroids; this was reversible upon withdrawal of the drug.

Temporary reduction in the function of the adrenal cortex (the source of the body's cortisone) is common following withdrawal of prolonged corticosteroid treatment. This is probably secondary to a suppression of the pituitary gland by the medication. And since the pituitary controls the adrenal, suppression of the former causes the latter to slow down or cease its function. Symptoms are very similar to those seen in the disease caused by adrenal gland insufficiency, Addison's Disease. There is headache, weakness, loss of appetite, pain in joints and muscles, and excessive fatigue. Short courses of corticosteroids will not cause this phenomenon. Prolonged high dosage, however, may require up to six months for the pituitary adrenal network to repair itself and get back into full action. And indeed there are some of us who feel that the adrenal cortex may remain relatively injured for the rest of the patient's life. This means that it functions normally during the minor physiological stresses of day-to-day living: But if the human organism is subjected to a severely stressful situation (traumatic auto accident, major surgery, catastrophic medical illness), the adrenal may not be able to respond optimally.

There have been some instances of mysterious irreversible shock occurring in patients undergoing major surgery. Subsequent history disclosed that these patients had received prolonged, high-dose corticosteroid therapy at some time in the past. Under such circumstances one must provide the patient with supplemental corticosteroids to tide him over the period of crisis. In anticipation of major surgery, we give "prophylactic" corticosteroids to the patient who is known to have received corticosteroids in high dosage for prolonged periods at a former time.

Many other adverse effects have been attributed to corticosteroids, but we have discussed the major ones.

Thus the period of the pendulum has taken its characteristic course. The swing goes from initial enthusiasm→widespread undisciplined clinical use→unanticipated adverse effects→panicky withdrawal→publication of results of work done by careful investigators (started during "initial enthusiasm")→careful reflection and reappraisal of drug efficacy and toxicity→drug slides into place as a valuable (but not entirely benign) agent.

In the case of the corticosteroids, its amazing spectrum of utility maintains its place high on the list of contemporary "wonder drugs." But it has taken about twenty years for it to fall into proper perspective, where its efficacy and toxicity are fully appreciated and respected.

If the current climate of drug discovery persists, one must conclude that "Diseases of Medical Progress" will be with us forevermore. They cannot be swept under the rug, either by clinician or drug producer.

My own naïveté in the world of commercial enterprise is revealed by my admission that I think a fine new drug will become known to the profession on the basis of its merit. I am embarrassed when this noble commodity is demeaned by merchandising techniques, however subtle or artful, better suited to less vital products, such as soap or soda pop. I do not feel that drugs should be propagandized to the medical profession. The pressure of commercial competition is not conducive to objectivity in the presentations of drug detail men or in published advertisements. I feel these factors add to the confusion in the already difficult problems of evaluating the efficacy and/or adverse effects of new drugs.

The requirement for an impartial agency that can provide current, reliable, and objective data about the characteristics of new drugs and alert the physician to their toxic hazards is abundantly evident. This requirement has now been met by the American Medical Association Council on Drugs, which created a national "Registry of Adverse Reactions." This broad registry makes it possible for any physician to contribute his personal experience with adverse drug effects to a central pool. Such information is recorded on a form designed for automatic data processing. The data are extracted and recorded in the memory banks of a computer system.

Volunteer teams of nationally recognized specialists study all information submitted to the Registry. Thus the input from physicians throughout the country is evaluated and recorded. At hand, for the first time, are the means for obtaining realistic incidence data about adverse drug effects. The program is young, but already *The Journal of the American Medical Association* has carried many brief, pertinent articles describing recently discovered adverse drug effects and summarizing experiences derived from this new facility.

The Federal Drug Administration has inaugurated a similar program that complements the American Medical Association Registry and expands the total data-gathering capability. Federal Drug Administration concern in the matter is oriented somewhat differently from that of the American Medical Association. Nevertheless, such activity in the nation's highest medical councils indicates the growing importance of adverse drug effects.

The American Medical Association Registry represents a significant step toward meeting the challenge of new responsibility that accompanies our increased capability. Our remarkable therapeutic arsenal is a tribute to the commercial drug industry and the devoted chemists and pharmacologists of our medical schools. But neither the schools, the AMA, the FDA, nor the industry can solve the problem completely.

My plea has been, and is directed to the physician on the firing line: the doctor who prescribes the drug. It is furthest from my intention to suggest therapeutic timidity or homeopathy.

Our predecessors in medicine had limited diagnostic and therapeutic resources. The complement of nostrums in their little black bag was austere, but these drugs were regarded as old, familiar friends. Some were worthless, others dangerous; some were impure and unstandardized to the point of unpredictability. The few effective drugs were trusted allies whose strengths and weaknesses were well known. The practitioner of the past attempted to compensate for lack of material resources with meticulous attention to his patients, personal charm, kindness, and pervading equanimity.

His lonely hours of private hell, tormented by his inability to come to grips with most of the severe illnesses he encountered, constitute a long, bleak chapter in the chronicle of medicine. The modern physician is afforded rarer glimpses of this agony, as when faced with malignancy or degenerative disease or certain neurologic illnesses. Modern pharmacology has brought this unhappy era nearer to an end; we now enjoy the privilege of fine, powerful, well-standardized therapeutic weapons.

Now we must work to create an atmosphere of rational caution and critical evaluation, where each physician will pause before putting pen to prescription pad and ask himself, "Do I know enough about this drug to prescribe it? Does the possible benefit I hope to derive from this drug outweigh its potential hazard?"

I do not preach therapeutic nihilism, but rather, therapeutic rationalism.

NOTE ON CONTRIBUTOR

Robert H. Moser, Colonel, MC, USA, (M.D., Georgetown University, 1948) is chief of the Medical Service at Brooke General Hospital, Fort Sam Houston, Texas. He also is assigned to the manned spacecraft program, serving the Mercury, Gemini, and Apollo missions. He was a research fellow in pulmonary disease at the (Washington) D.C. General Hospital in 1949-1950 and a research fellow in hematology, Salt Lake County Hospital, Utah. He is on the editorial board of several medical journals and contributes a monthly column to *Clinical Pharmacology and Therapeutics* and is the author of *Diseases of Medical Progress*. He has been a member of the advisory panel of the Registry of Adverse Reactions, Council on Drugs of the American Medical Association since 1960.

Fig 9: Examples of Ventricular Hypertrophy.

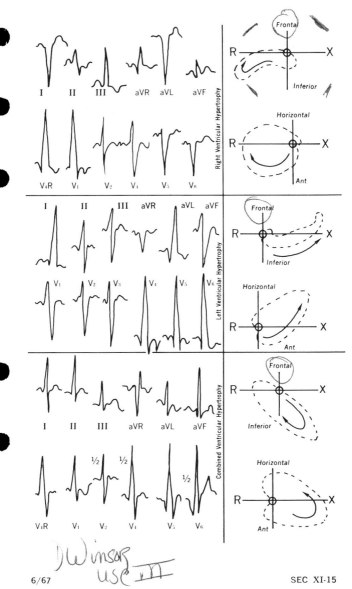

I II III aVR aVL aVF

V₄R V₁ V₂ V₄ V₅ V₆

Right Ventricular Hypertrophy

I II III aVR aVL aVF

V₁ V₂ V₃ V₄ V₅ V₆

Left Ventricular Hypertrophy

I II III aVR aVL aVF

V₄R V₁ V₂ V₄ V₅ V₆

Combined Ventricular Hypertrophy

Frontal
R ——— X
Inferior

Horizontal
R ——— X
Ant

Fig 8a: Normal Progression of Frontal mean QRS axis in Frontal Plane VCG and key limb leads.

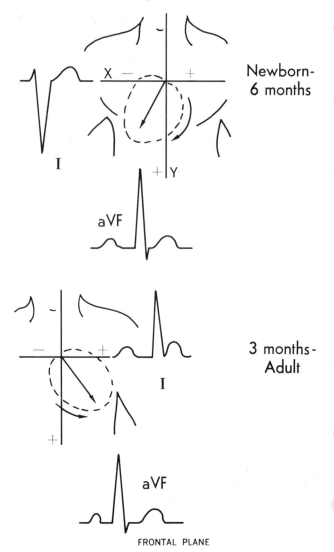

Newborn-
6 months

3 months-
Adult

FRONTAL PLANE

10

Science Versus Ethics in Human Drug Trials: Problems and Solutions

THOMAS C. CHALMERS, M.D.

THIS TITLE IMPLIES a conflict between science and ethics in clinical investigation. The theme I shall present is that no conflict should exist or develop in this field of endeavor, because the clinical investigator is a physician, and there can be no argument that the physician's primary responsibility is for the welfare of his patient. In recognition of that responsibility he must live by the motto *primum non nocere* (first do no harm), but he must also be willing to admit his lack of adequate knowledge about how best to treat most of the ills now plaguing mankind. To correct this lack requires scientific investigation, and the patient who is the subject of a new drug study might well fare better than the patient treated by an "established" drug that some day may be proved worthless or even harmful. In addition, the meticulous screening of patients taking part in the trial of experimental drugs can be expected to result in excellent general medical care.

Webster's first definition of science is "the possession of

knowledge as distinguished from ignorance or misunderstanding." Ethics is defined as "the discipline dealing with what is good and bad, and with moral duty and obligation." I shall try to show that drug trials in man not only can but must satisfy the requirements implied by both definitions.

In order best to explain the interplay of science and ethics in human research and the implications of such technical details as the use of controls, the obtaining of *informed* consent, and the protection of volunteers, it will be worthwhile to outline the development of a new drug from the laboratory to the physician's prescription pad. To do this I shall invent an imaginary drug for a very real disease. I shall concentrate on describing how human trials of this new drug can and should be considered a part of the best possible practice of medicine, as well as being modestly thought of as a part of science.

Obviously a need for a new drug must exist before an effort is made to evaluate its effects in man. The drug must be of potential benefit to its consumer rather than primarily to its manufacturer, advertiser, or clinical investigator.

The need for new and better drugs in most of medical practice is so obvious that one is belaboring a point to recite them, but I shall do so to offer a frame of reference for what is to come. In every field of medicine we not only need drugs to eliminate disease processes, that is to prevent or cure, but we also need improved drugs to alleviate symptoms. To start with the killer diseases, we need drugs to prevent premature atherosclerosis. We need drugs that will prevent and cure cancer, not just the currently available drugs that make the tumor shrink. We need drugs that will prevent the process leading to elevation of the blood pressure and rupture of vital blood vessels, not just drugs that lower the pressure without necessarily reversing the basic process.

Drugs aimed at the killer diseases will merely prolong life; what we really need are better drugs to prolong health, to prevent and treat disabling disease. The greatest cause of time lost from work, or of hospitalization in diagnostic centers, is not one of the killer diseases, but rather digestive and respiratory disorders. We need better drugs for treating the estimated three and one-half million people in this country who were affected by peptic ulcers during 1965. We need drugs to help control the diarrheal diseases that impair the health of so much of the world's population. Commonly available drugs only partially relieve the symptoms of the three million people with arthritis in this country. No drugs safely stop the inflammatory process that gradually destroys the joints in patients with arthritis, or scars the liver in patients with cirrhosis. We can only treat the symptoms of patients with these diseases. It is possible that mental illnesses will some day be prevented or successfully treated by drugs, but we need more effective ones than are now available.

Some day drugs will be found that can accomplish these "medical miracles." Before they can be established as both efficacious and safe, however, they will have to be given to volunteers and to patients with the appropriate disease, utilizing clinical trials that are both scientific and ethical.

Let us review the steps that might be taken in the development of a new drug for one of the above—say the specific treatment of peptic ulcer. There is no doubt about the need. Besides the disability referred to above, over twelve thousand people in the United States die of peptic ulcer disease each year. Rather drastic surgery has been variably fashionable. No one denies that a safe medical or drug "cure" would be preferable, but none exists. We can only treat the symptoms, and there is some doubt about the comparative efficacy of available drugs in accomplishing that.

Let us imagine that a physician employed by a pharmaceutical firm learns from his children studying American Indians that a certain tribe habitually chewed the bark of old birch canoes whenever they had "belly distress." He wisely notes that this was an unwarlike tribe, one harassed by other tribes in the area, yet one in which it was essential for the male to maintain his superiority in the eyes of the female without committing overt aggression—*i.e.,* the men must have had peptic ulcers and have chewed birch bark for relief. And they must have preferred old canoes to fresh bark because prolonged soaking improved the efficacy of the substance (drug) or removed some toxic substance (side effect). A multimillion-dollar research program was promptly launched by our imaginary pharmaceutical house.

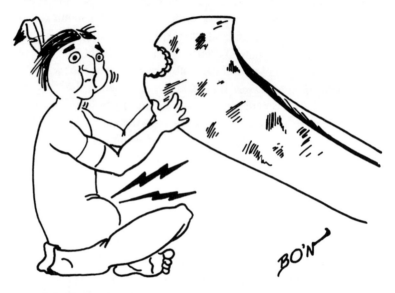

Animal models are only partially available for the development of drugs active against peptic ulcer. Effects on normal gastric function can be studied, and ulcers can be created, but only under quite abnormal circumstances. As in man, however, peptic ulcers are never found in the absence of acid. Let us assume that BBCE (birch bark canoe extract) was found to cause lasting atrophy of acid-secreting cells in dogs, and thus to be a highly promising anti-ulcer medication. Short- and long-term toxicity studies in various species of animals revealed it to have no other demonstrable effects in doses many times that necessary to eliminate acid secretion. No fetal abnormalities were demonstrable in pregnant animals taking the drug. The active principle was isolated and identified, and an economically feasible synthesis was devised. Patent proceedings were begun. An **IND** (investigation of new drug) application was submitted to the Food and Drug Administration, and accompanying this were all of the toxicity data and protocols for initial trials in men, literally pounds of information.

As Pope has said "the proper study of mankind is man."

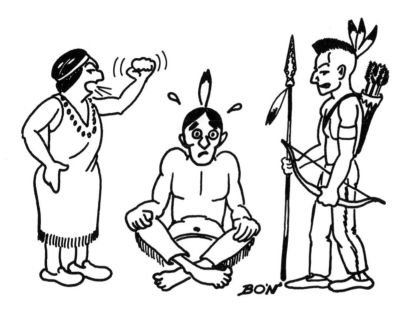

BBCE was ready for trial in humans. The four stages of that trial offer us a framework in which to discuss the ethical problems raised.

PHASE I: INITIAL TRIAL FOR PRELIMINARY INFORMATION REGARDING DOSAGE, METABOLISM, GOOD EFFECTS, AND TOXICITY

This state of a new drug development is usually carried out in volunteers, people without the disease to be treated. They may be employees of the institution, local students, or inhabitants of a prison. The scientific aspects of this phase involve the design and execution of a sophisticated pharmacologic study, one in which all possible toxic effects are searched for, as well as the effects on gastric function. Since no animal accurately predicts the response of a man to drugs, dosage and duration of administration must be

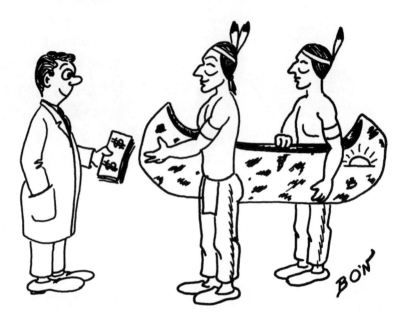

increased very slowly. Accurate techniques for measuring absorption, metabolism, excretion, and pharmacological effects may have to be outlined.

In the case of BBCE the volunteers had to swallow tubes frequently to determine the effects on gastric acid secretion. In moderate doses the drug was effective for many months, and the only apparent side effect was tingling of the fingers and soreness of the tongue of a few medical student volunteers, an effect not found among the less well-informed prisoners.

The ethical aspects of Phase I studies revolve around the selection and protection of healthy volunteers. It is useless to argue, as some have, about the ultimate freedom of choice of the volunteer. Whether the sacrifice is a minor discomfort or expenditure of time, or a threat to health or life, no matter how rare, each individual has something to gain from volunteering, which to him makes up for the risk. It may be money, the satisfaction of helping mankind, something to boast about, a credit with the boss, a possibly profitable friendship with the investigator, or the hope, although it can only be a hope, of a more favorable review by the parole board. At any rate the volunteer must be fully informed of the discomfort and risk, as far as is known at the time, so he can make a rational decision. At the same time the investigator must make every effort to avoid any semblance of coercion in obtaining volunteers.

The investigator, and his peers who are responsible for approving the study, must be confident that the research is important to the health of man, that it must be carried out in humans, and that the approach is sound from the scientific standpoint. To satisfy these requirements all institutions carrying out research in humans have committees that must pass on protocols and the suitability of procedures outlined for informing the volunteer or patient and obtaining his permission. Such committees should include, in addition to experienced investigators, practicing physicians and occasionally interested laymen.

As soon as an investigator *tests* a volunteer, he also becomes the man's physician. When the investigator is not a skilled clinician, the volunteer must have a second doctor to look after his health during and after the research project.

It has been suggested that the patient's physician serve as the "friendly adversary" of the investigator, the defender of the patient. In our teaching hospitals the medical students, interns, and residents, who are learning to be good doctors, and the attending physicians who are teaching them, admirably fulfill that function.

The health of the volunteer is protected by the adequacy of animal-screening procedures (never entirely satisfactory), by the experience of the responsible pharmacologists in predicting effects from chemical structure, and by the skill and caution of the physician-investigator. He needs one more protection, compensation insurance, a very excellent suggestion made by Irving Ladimer, a lawyer and consultant to the United States Public Health Service, who has given many years to developing a functional legal attitude toward clinical investigation. Mr. Ladimer has advocated a plan that has not been accepted as readily as I think it should have been. At present a volunteer who suffers an untoward or unexpected reaction, one requiring loss of time from work or hospitalization, must rely on the good will of the investigator to arrange compensation, or must sue the investigator as if an unethical act, malpractice, or illegal assault had been committed. Investigators should carry a form of insurance similar in concept to workmen's compensation insurance, which will allow for recompense on the basis of an unpreventable side effect of the research, rather than requiring litigation based on an assumed fault or negligence. Compensation of the volunteer who suffers from an unexpected complication of the research would thus not be based on a fault, if any, on the part of the investigator or those who approved the trial, but rather on the assumed risk that an adverse effect could occur. Such insurance is in effect a cost of doing the business of research, just as premiums for work-injury insurance are part of the usual industrial or commercial cost. Details of such an insurance plan may be difficult to work out, and there may be disadvantages not readily apparent, but it is clear that the idea should be thoroughly explored.

PHASE II: DISEASE SPECIFIC TRIAL: TO ESTIMATE
BENEFICIAL AND TOXIC EFFECTS AT VARYING DOSAGE
IN THE SPECTRUM OF DISEASES IN WHICH
THE DRUG MAY BE USED

Phase II is really an extension of Phase I, and the two may overlap or blend together, since pharmacological data will continue to be carefully gathered in the diseased patients. Several definitions are necessary here to clarify both the scientific and the ethical aspects of the trial of a new drug in humans with a disease, both in Phase II and III trials.

Random assignment means that the decision as to whether the patient receives the new drug or not is made by chance; that is the selection is not made according to the medical indications in that particular patient. The need for and justification of this technique will become clear as we learn how the efficacy of birch bark canoe extract is established.

Controls are the patients who are treated in exactly the same manner as those who receive the new drugs except that they receive the standard or best-known therapy instead. If no effective therapy is available, they may be given a *placebo,* or sugar pill, to take advantage of the psychic effects of medication. The use of controls in a drug trial allows the detection of both good and bad effects, which might falsely have been attributed to the drug if the comparison group were not available.

A *double-blind study* is one in which neither the patient nor the physician knows, at the time of administration and at the time of evaluation of the drug's effect in the individual, whether or not he received the active principle.

Each of these four techniques, as will be shown by the example of BBCE, may be essential components of the scientifically valid trial. They are also entirely ethical tools of the physician-investigator, provided it is entirely clear to both him and his peers who approve the research that *it is not known* whether the patient who receives the active drug or the control patient will benefit more from the doctor's treatment. The ethical justification for the controlled trial rests not on the *ignorance* of physicians, but rather on their *knowledge* that they do not have the information necessary to decide how to treat the patient, although they realize that some treatment must be effected.

There are two major distinctions to be kept in mind when a

patient with a disease, other than a normal volunteer, is given a new drug.

• Trials in the patient with disease are always fraught with the danger that an effect of the disease may be misinterpreted by the patient and the investigator as a side effect, or vice versa. A classic example is the comment many years ago of a patient who had been saved by penicillin when on the brink of death due to lobar pneumonia; "That new drug may be life-saving but it certainly leaves you feeling washed out." The patient had no insight into the fact that he might feel washed out because he had been so deathly ill. Many of the chemotherapeutic drugs now being used in patients with tumors depress the bone marrow or immune mechanisms exactly as some tumors do, and it may be hard to distinguish drug from disease effects. That is why randomly assigned controls are usually necessary for Phase II studies. Such an assignment is entirely ethical because the drug is being prescribed without prior knowledge as to whether it will be more helpful than harmful.

• Secondly, it should be recognized that a patient with a disease to be treated is seldom a volunteer. Occasionally he is sought out by an investigator and agrees to be studied for reasons similar to those of healthy volunteers, but usually he takes part in a study because he has more to gain than to lose with regard to his own health. This brings us to one of the *most important* points I have to make. When an investigator in a Phase II study gives a new drug to a patient with a symptom or a disease to be treated, he must be convinced that the patient has more to gain than to lose by taking part in the trial. Sick patients have enough to worry about without being urged to volunteer for studies of a drug that could *only* make them sicker. So the physician must have some knowledge, or at least a hunch, that people with the disease who are first given a new drug will be favorably affected. This does not obviate the need for a scientific dose response study in which small and large doses are compared. This must be done first when the proper dose in man has not yet been determined. If the drug turns out to be more toxic than useful, the patient who received the small dose by chance will benefit most. If the drug is nontoxic and effective only in large amounts, the patient receiving a high dose will be the lucky one.

As in the case of the volunteer, the benefit to the subject himself must be commensurate with the risk. When the trial of a new drug is being considered, the investigator must have reason to think that it may have distinct advantages over conventional treatment, or he must not use it. From the ethical as well as the legal standpoint he cannot pursue the investigation of a drug he has reason to fear is worse than conventional treatment. Of course, the rub here is that firm opinions about efficacy and toxicity require carefully executed scientific drug trials, *i.e.,* usually Phase III studies as described below. But before we get into them, let's briefly follow the progress of BBCE through Phase II trials.

Several clinics specializing in gastrointestinal disease, especially those equipped to carry out studies of gastric physiology in humans, were contacted by our mythical pharmaceutical company. Protocols were prepared, approved by local human research committees, and forwarded to the Food and Drug Administration. The acute effects of the drug on gastric secretion were then studied and administration was continued longer than in the Phase I volunteers to determine the effects of varying doses.

What are the potential benefits and dangers to the patient with peptic ulcer who is about to receive this new drug? As indicated above, the disease is a nasty one. Although most acute attacks respond to conservative therapy, the relapse rate is high, and life-threatening complications may require surgery or result in death, or both. So a drug that cures the disease at little risk may well be worth a try to the average patient. In the sense that suitable dosage regimens are worked out from information gained during his treatment, he is a volunteer. But his only reward is treatment of his disease, and an abnormal effect of the drug should be regarded as a complication of the treatment of the disease, as with any other treatment. The patient accepts the risk when he accepts the treatment, but in this case he puts his fate in the hands of his doctor as an investigator as well as a physician. It is possible that research compensation insurance should also apply to patients taking part in Phase II trials, but many problems would be introduced by the difficulty one might encounter in distinguishing between the effects of the disease and those of the new drug.

PHASE III: THE CONTROLLED CLINICAL TRIAL: COMPARISON OF THE NEW DRUG WITH THE BEST KNOWN MEDICAL THERAPY, WITH OR WITHOUT A PLACEBO

After an apparently effective dosage regimen had been worked out and prohibitive toxicity ruled out, BBCE was ready for a definitive trial. Remember the definitions of *random assignment, controls, placebo,* and *double-blind study* given above. Here the random assignment to treated and control groups would be essential to all trials, and the use of a suitable control medication and double-blinding would be necessary in all those in which a comparative evaluation of drug effects and toxicity is being made.

Why is the use of *controls* so important to the proper interpretation of drug effects in patients? For one thing it is essential to be able to separate coincidental occurrences in the course of the disease from the effects of the drug. Whenever students are too ready to assume that something prescribed for the patient caused an effect that might have been coincidental, I remind them of the "Bathtub in the Blitz." During World War II, at the time of the London blitz, a great teacher of mine, Dr. David Seegal of Columbia, arrived at work excitedly waving a copy of the morning *Times.* In it was a factual account of the experience of rescue workers digging in the ruins of an apartment house that had been blown up the day before. An old man was found lying naked in a bathtub, fully conscious.

"You know," he said to his rescuers, "that was the most amazing experience I ever had. When I pulled the plug and the water started down the drain, the whole house blew up."

A second purpose of controls is to enable the physician-investigator to distinguish between the natural history of the untreated

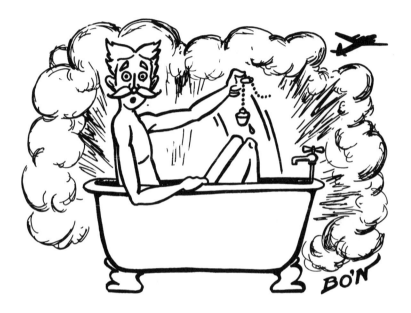

disease and the effects of the drug. Many diseases are self-limited and uninfluenced by therapy. They are also extremely variable in duration. This variability of disease, and of patients' response to it, is at the same time the most fascinating and frustrating aspect of medical practice. How does the physician determine whether or not a drug given to a patient with a self-limiting disease of variable duration is responsible for his ultimate improvement? In practice, and unfortunately in many clinical trials of drugs, physicians try one therapy after another until one works, or the patient tries a new doctor. My father-in-law, a layman, once pointed out to me that "the last ointment you put on your poison ivy is *always* the one that works." Only by comparison with randomly assigned controls can the effects of the drug be distinguished from the natural history of the disease.

This brings us to another important technique of the controlled drug trial: the determination of both direct and side-effects without knowledge of whether the patient is receiving an active or inactive agent (double-blinding). Many patients are able to take a potentially toxic drug without any abnormal symptoms. Some patients develop all sorts of symptoms on a placebo. Asking for symptoms frequently brings them out. Remember the sensitive, and generally sensible man whose fellow office workers laid a trap for him on April first. It was a beautiful day and he arrived at work feeling fine. But the first man he greeted asked if he felt all right. The next said he looked a little pale. Someone else asked if he had been up all night. The plot continued, and by noon he felt sick enough to call a doctor.

The only way to determine whether a drug improves or worsens the symptoms of a disease is to control the biases and suggestibility of both patient and physician by double-blinding the observations. But this constitutes manipulation of a sick patient for the purposes of research, and that we have agreed is unethical *unless* it is in the best interests of the individual patient. The following discussion is intended to show that the trial in which blinding is essential to the proper interpretation of symptoms is in the best interests of the patient who is lucky enough to take part in it.

We are often told that no controls were necessary to demonstrate the efficacy of quinine in malaria, insulin in diabetes, liver extract in pernicious anemia, or penicillin in pneumonia. But these are just four of the many thousands of drugs on the market. Many others, introduced without a controlled trial, were used for years before doctors decided that they really did more harm than good. Benjamin Rush, one of the most famous physicians of eighteenth-century America, vigorously bled and purged patients dying of yellow fever in Philadelphia, absolutely the worst possible treatment, but no one appreciated that at the time. A control group of patients might have lived instead of died, as well as have saved the lives of future patients by demonstrating that the treatment was harmful. There are many modern examples of dangerous drugs, which might have been detected and withdrawn much sooner had scientific trials been carried out from the beginning.

An equally disturbing example of the need for a controlled trial is the danger that a potentially useful drug will be withdrawn from the market because of a dramatic but infrequent side effect. One of the early drugs introduced to combat depression was thought without a controlled trial to prevent suicide. With widespread usage it became apparent that approximately one in two thousand patients developed hepatitis and one in ten thousand died of that disease. On the basis of this toxicity the drug was withdrawn. Subsequently introduced less toxic drugs may or may not be as effective.

It has been estimated that six thousand people commit suicide each year in the United States as the result of a mental depression. If ten depressed patients had to be treated for every suicidal one, there might have been, among sixty thousand depressed people treated, thirty cases of hepatitis and approximately six fatalities. On the other hand the drug might have prevented 10 per cent of the six thousand from committing suicide or prevented six hundred deaths, at a loss of six. This is an admirable therapeutic-toxicity ratio, especially in view of the fact that many of the sixty thousand might have benefited symptomatically.

All of this speculation about possibly needless deaths or premature removal of a drug could have been avoided if a large-scale, properly controlled trial had been carried out as soon as clinical usefulness and safety of the drug was suspected. Assume the same figures as above; there might have been three more fatalities from hepatitis and three hundred *less* suicides in the thirty thousand given the drug, and probably less disability than in the thirty thousand treated with conventional therapy plus a placebo. The saving of so many lives might have been well worth the risk of hepatitis, but such a trial would have had to be carried out before inaccurate prejudices could develop about the drug's good and bad effects. The drug had to be withdrawn because it apparently caused hepatitis, when no reliable information was available as to whether or not it prevented suicide. Incidentally, it is still on the market in England.

Let me review the principles of the therapeutic trial by returning to BBCE, our potential answer to the dyspeptic's prayer. In the Phase II studies it became apparent that BBCE, like most other drugs, had a beneficial effect in most but not all patients, and some toxicity, but the relative frequency and importance of the good and bad effects were unknown. Two courses of action were open to interested physicians. They could gradually and cautiously increase their experience with the drug and try to weigh the benefit versus the risk, or they could begin a large-scale trial, possibly a cooperative one, as soon as Phase II studies suggested the best regimen. Such a trial would compare BBCE with usual medical and surgical therapy plus a placebo, with the patients carefully selected and then randomly assigned to each treatment.

Let us illustrate the importance of the latter course by assuming that, heaven forbid, BBCE is tried extensively in an uncontrolled fashion by two large gastrointestinal clinics. One concludes that the drug is much better than surgery for patients with peptic ulcer, and the other concludes that surgery is much better. How could this happen? The patients referred to the two clinics were similar, the dosage regimen and the methods of measuring treatment effect were the same. The explanation lay in the orientation of the physicians of the two clinics with regard to the efficacy of surgery, in this case the control regimen. One clinic was a vigorous proponent of medical treatment and referred only the most difficult cases to the surgeon. The patients selected by them for BBCE did very well, when compared with those who had surgery because their disease was considered too far advanced for medical therapy. The other clinic was dominated by surgeons who firmly believed that surgery had more to offer ulcer patients than medical therapy. They felt that they could not deprive the young patient with early disease of the benefits of curative surgery. So they tried the new drug only on the "surgery rejects," and as might be expected, encountered more toxicity and less therapeutic effects than the investigators who gave it to their "best" patients. This is not an apocryphal story. Examples abound in the medical literature. In each instance it is impossible to separate, after the fact, the effects of treatment from those of selection of the patient for that treatment.

Let's imagine we are going to avoid that tragic mistake in the evaluation of BBCE. A scientific trial would be worked out by competent gastroenterologists, pharmacologists, and biostatisticians. The protocol would be approved by committees of their peers, and by their chiefs of service. Patients with demonstrated recurrent ulcers would be selected for the study and randomly assigned to treatment and control groups. The end points to be compared would be permanent disappearance of symptoms and prevention of complications requiring surgery. Would the random assignment of patients with acute peptic ulcers to BBCE or a placebo, in a double-blind trial, be an ethical way to treat such patients? As a start, we must be humble and honest enough to recognize our ignorance, or rather our need for knowledge. We do not know whether on the average the good effects of the drug, elimination of acid secretion in the stomach and thus of peptic ulcer, will be more than outweighed by the bad effects, be they simply troublesome or life-threatening. We don't know the frequency of these contrasting effects in different ages, sex, or genetic backgrounds. Thus we cannot predict in any given patient the effects of the drug or the outcome of the untreated disease.

We have presented potent scientific arguments against the conduct of an indefinite uncontrolled trial. Is it ethical to withhold this drug from patients with peptic ulcer because we do not *know* that it is effective and has few short or long-term side-effects?

Isn't inaction as potentially unethical as action, when neither is based on essential knowledge, referred to in medical circles as *the data?* Obviously the best chance for the patient is to be part of a controlled trial when one is available, because then he will have a fifty-fifty chance of receiving the right treatment, and whichever he draws he will probably be observed much more carefully than the patient treated in a routine fashion. This is especially so in the trial under question, because it is assumed that BBCE or a placebo will be added to the standard therapy of an acute ulcer, such as diet and antacids.

So it can be argued that it is unethical *not* to persuade a patient to enter a controlled trial when a potentially beneficial treatment is available but has not yet been proved to be more efficacious than toxic. If it should turn out that the drug causes more harm than good, the patient given a placebo will be better off than the one who received the active principle, and he could also be better off than the patient who received nothing, and thus less medical attention.

One very important moral principle needs to be emphasized here. If a physician *thinks* he knows whether or not a treatment will, on the average, benefit a particular patient, it is unethical for him to encourage or allow that patient to enter a controlled trial of the new treatment. This is the one reason why so many drugs used today have never been established as efficacious by a properly controlled trial. Physicians are loath to admit to themselves or to their patients that they really don't know whether a drug is harmful or beneficial. They may not have been as critical of the existing therapeutic trial literature as they should have been, or they may actually conduct an uncontrolled trial of a new drug under the mistaken impression that it is more ethical than a controlled trial. It is remarkable how many investigators of new drugs have made this mistake.

A physician who may have been convinced that a controlled trial was indicated for a given patient cannot keep that patient in the trial if his clinical judgment tells him that the clinical trial is preventing the patient from receiving an apparently better treatment. *Primum non nocere:* This is an important safety factor in any trial. But the physician must have a firm basis for his clinical decision to withdraw the patient.

PHASE IV: FIELD TRIALS: THE MONITORED USE OF NEW AND OLD DRUGS IN THE CLINICAL PRACTICE OF MEDICINE

The uncontrolled trial of new drugs by physicians whose primary function is the practice of medicine is considered by some, including the Food and Drug Administration, to be a part of Phase III. However, the use of controls is so essential to proper evaluation of new drugs that only the controlled trial should be included in Phase III. After that has demonstrated sufficient usefulness to suggest that the drug might be marketed, distribution to practicing physicians is carried out to obtain further information about its usefulness "in the field." Here, such aspects as ease of administration and patient acceptability are evaluated, and information is accumulated about possible side effects too rare to be picked up by the usual controlled clinical trial. These clinical observations should continue long after the release of the drug for general use. Is a new disease going to develop in patients whose acid-secreting cells have been destroyed by BBCE? Alert practicing physicians will detect this if it occurs. Similarly, there is a great need for the recording of toxic effects of all drugs used in practice, but this information is useless without accurate data on drug usage and the ratio of toxic to desirable effects in the routine practice of medicine. All practicing physicians should be more active in the *systematic* recording of both the good and bad effects of drugs. This is one way in which highly beneficial research can be introduced into routine practice. No "manipulation" of the patient is required, just the recording of data in a way in which it can be analyzed.

One important and new aspect of drug trials in man is just

emerging, namely the detection of good or bad effects due to combinations of drugs administered to the same patient. Most hospitalized patients receive many drugs, and we are only beginning to learn in experimental animals and man how one drug may seriously affect the metabolism of another. Clues to these phenomena can only be picked up by the careful monitoring of drug usage. We are in great need of much more information on the interaction of drugs, and all physicians must be investigators if this need is to be met.

There should be no ethical problems in Phase IV trials. The physician who uses new or old drugs under monitoring circumstances is actually being more responsible to his patients than at any other time in his practice.

These concluding points will summarize what has been said above. First, the trial of a new drug should not be considered as something ethically apart from the routine practice of medicine. Doctors frequently use officially approved medicines that may be toxic and have never been established as efficacious. They don't obtain written permission to do so. I suspect that it is still not known whether the majority of drugs used today are more or less effective or harmful than other drugs in the same category, or than no drug therapy. Does this mean that it is less ethical to use, or to withhold, such previously approved drugs?

The second point has to do with the difficult-to-define requirement of informed consent. This is a legal term that doctors have begun to use widely, while at the same time admitting that they are unclear about its exact definition. Does a patient need to know *everything* about his disease and the new therapy before he allows the physician to treat him as part of a new drug trial? Here there is an important distinction between the volunteer who is given a drug primarily for research purposes and only secondarily for his own benefit, and the patient who receives a drug primarily to treat his disease and secondarily for research purposes. Consent should be explicit in the first instance; it should, in the judgment of the physician, be qualified in the second instance.

The art of medicine requires that the good physician tell the patient what it seems best for him to know, frankly and honestly discussing the disease and its treatment, old or experimental. If it seems in the best interests of the patient to receive a new drug, the physician should not be required to be brutal in his frankness, simply because regulations or fear of a lawsuit require brutality when a new drug is being used and not when an old one is being used.

It also can be argued that it is not good medical practice to explain to a patient every scientific detail that goes into a decision to give or withhold a particular drug. Physicians are well informed about the hazards of various diseases and the possible side effects of treatment. They make terrible patients. The physician who treats himself has a fool for a doctor because he is too personally involved to make rational decisions. It follows that it might not be in the best interest of all patients to try to make them as informed as a physician-patient of the hazards they face.

Speaking as a layman in the legal sense, I should say that it would be most important for a physician to be able to establish, for the sake of his conscience, the approval of his peers, the authorities regulating the study of new drugs, and any future court of law, that he acted in the best interests of his patient by trying a drug that had at least a good chance of directly benefiting the patient, according to a protocol that had been found to be scientifically and ethically acceptable. "Informed" consent for the performance of an unscientific or unethical procedure could be obtained with ease by an unconscientious physician. It is more important to equate the trial of new drugs with the practice of medicine; the physician should always be able to establish that he acted in the best interests of his patient.

Finally, great good has come out of the inquiry carried out in the last few years into the ethical aspects of scientific research in humans. Inevitably the rights and comforts of the patients will be considered more seriously, and the setting up of standards of scientific excellence and of committees of peers to approve all research protocols is sure to improve the quality of clinical research, while at the same time protecting both the patient and the physician-investigator.

NOTE ON CONTRIBUTOR

Thomas C. Chalmers is chief of Medical Services, Lemuel Shattuck Hospital, and professor of medicine, Tufts University School of Medicine, Boston, Massachusetts. He was graduated from Columbia College of Physicians and Surgeons, 1943. He directed the hepatitis study for the Commission on Liver Disease of the Armed Forces Epidemiological Board, and served on the Cancer Chemotherapy Collaborative Program Review Committee for the National Cancer Institute. Presently he is a member of several national committees, including: the Special Projects Committee of the National Heart Institute; National Academy of Sciences-National Research Council, Committee on Epidemiological and Veterans Follow-Up Studies; the Surgeon-General's Advisory Committee on General Medicine, subcommittee on the liver; American Public Health Association's Committee on New Drugs; and the Scientific Advisory Committee of the Pharmaceutical Manufacturers Association Foundation.

11

The Contributions of the
Pharmaceutical Industry

CHESTER S. KEEFER, M.D.

WHEN MEN ENTERED medicine half a century ago, many felt helpless in the face of sick people. It was a depressing situation to watch women dying of childbed fever; many dying of pneumonia, influenza, meningitis, tuberculosis, septicemia, diabetes, syphilis of the brain and vascular system, or being crippled by poliomyelitis.

Today the situation is different because of the advance of science and therapeutics, and the development of new drugs, vaccines, and antitoxins. But much remains to be done.

It is difficult for those who have not lived through this period to have a full appreciation of the changes that have taken place, and it is more difficult for many to share my enthusiasm as a physician about drugs and their benefits to mankind.

In fact, in some quarters the climate of public opinion is cool to say the least about all of the health professions and especially with regard to drugs, their development and use. To some, the word drug or medicine has acquired almost a derogatory tinge, sometimes called a nightmare.

In the minds of many and to some in very high places, drugs are immediately associated with physical deformities and new dread diseases, some of which may be fatal. Some consider drugs to be highly expensive and dangerous chemicals of dubious value with which our people are overdosed, and which are urged upon them or their doctors by the persuasive voice of commercial propaganda. As to drug manufacturers themselves and the scientific community within these industries, there are many—also in high places—who consider these professional scientists to be suspect; question their scientific judgment and integrity; and attempt to destroy public confidence in their work and what they are doing as professional men and the practitioners of science for humanity.

As a doctor, who has had an opportunity of observing the unfolding of new drugs over the past forty odd years and one who has studied these advances with high interest, I believe that drugs are one of man's greatest blessings, and as Professor Ernest Chain, the Nobel Laureate, has said, perhaps the greatest blessing of our time. Further, I have confidence in the scientific community and the health professions because of their achievements, and what they are doing for the benefit of society.

THE PHARMACEUTICAL INDUSTRY IN PERSPECTIVE

The modern pharmaceutical industry as viewed in perspective has a dual objective: First, to discover, develop, produce, and distribute drugs for the benefit of society; and second, to create social and economic gains under the present market system of the private economy. They do this through research and development of a discovery from the test tube to manufacture and distribution, so that medicine becomes available to meet the needs of human and animal health. They promote useful knowledge about their discoveries and products through the development of professional services to the health professions and the public. They do this in an effective manner by examining the needs and problems of their medical and pharmacy customers. They initiate support for postgraduate education, for medical and pharmacy schools themselves, for residents and interns and physicians just starting practice; they work with and seek to accommodate the needs of government agencies serving aid programs overseas or welfare programs in the United States; they underwrite health education activities of professional and voluntary health groups; they study the problems of hospitals and seek to aid in this difficult field. They cooperate in technological matters with academic, governmental, professional, and industrial institutions. They do this in pursuit of scientific and industry leadership, for the advancement of their organization, for the achievement of important business goals, and in so doing they engage in the pursuit of excellence.

Aside from meeting the needs of human and animal health through research, development, and promotion of useful knowledge about health and drugs, they create substantial economic and social gains under our present competitive market system. Here they create new markets, make investments around the world to improve the economy and health of all people. The economic performance of a company is of fundamental concern to its leaders and the public. The successful development and marketing of effective medicines is all within the framework of the private economy.

These dual motives of the industry serve as a stimulus to service and progress in the social and economic sense.

THE FUNCTION IN BRIEF OF THE
PHARMACEUTICAL INDUSTRY

Having stated the motives of the pharmaceutical industry, let me sketch momentarily how the prescription drug industry operates.

Those who are concerned with the affairs of this industry owe it to themselves to visit a modern pharmaceutical and biological research and production facility. The historical connotation of a slightly larger room at the back of the neighborhood apothecary shatters immediately as one steps into the halls of our leading firms. In them occur regular seminars, as in any school, or any of a thousand fine colleges. Drug company research seminars are not designed to mimic the academic world but to benefit from the same need to learn and to broaden intellectual horizons. Their research personnel now includes an estimated 16,000 sicentists and technical research people in the prescription drug industry. Each year their managements give them one-third of a billion dollars or approximately one million dollars a day to employ in the search for new and better medicines.

They work in *chemistry*—in physical, organic, and medicinal chemistry, and today pursue the micromolecular fields of DNA-RNA, polypeptides, and enzymes. They seek to relate the changes in the configuration of a chemical compound with its impact on the human organism, in the tradition of—but with fortunately much more knowledge than—Ehrlich seventy years ago, as he sought the "magic bullet" for target sites or target diseases.

They work with *microorganisms*—bacteria, viruses, fungi, and the cyclical existence of parasites; and they seek vaccines, as for polio, influenza, measles, mumps, and rubella.

They work with *animals*—mice, rats, monkeys, dogs, cats, pigs, chickens, horses—an estimated nine million of them a year. Each plays a role in finding out first whether the drug does anything to the living organism, and secondly whether it has toxic effects in the range of amounts necessary to achieve useful effects.

They work with *tissues*—the sections of organs and samples of blood that when examined show microscopically whether damage has been done and how much of the drug may be harmful, and what to look for if humans take too much.

They work in the skills of the apothecary, carried into the modern science of *pharmacy,* to prepare the chemical in a form the body can and will take, absorb, metabolize, and excrete—the capsule, the tablet, the solution or suspension or ointment.

Their laboratory work done, they turn to the clinics, medical centers, and physicians' offices for study of drugs in *humans*.

And when all the studies have been completed, they will ask approval of the Federal Food and Drug Administration to market the product for the uses that have been proved out by research.

From the basic chemical industry come raw materials to use in large-scale formulation of the new product. From the vast fermentation vats come antibiotics. In laboratorylike formulation facilities, the mixing, baking, compressing, coating, and other pharmaceutical processes take place, under the watchful eye of quality control inspectors. In the space-age-clean rooms of biological production, virus vaccines are grown, harvested, purified, and endlessly tested. From start to finish, statistical, numerical, procedural, physical, chemical, and analytical control systems attempt to reduce to near-zero the potential for error, mixup, distortion, or hazard.

Concurrently, a large group of well-informed men promote useful knowledge about the newly discovered drugs and provide information to doctors, pharmacists, and hospitals. This activity brings together the challenges of scientific professionalism and competitive marketing. But it is the responsibility of the industry to inform the profession and the public in the most professional, dignified, and effective manner about their products. The methods of communicating this information are improving in spite of the criticism that is leveled at them.

There are many reliable sources of information about drugs and their use, and new methods of communication are being developed by industry to ensure that all who use drugs have full information about them. Aside from the professional service personnel, sometimes called detail men because they are prepared to discuss the details of the drugs they talk about, information is available in the monographs published by the Council on Drugs of the American Medical Association, in the hundreds of medical journals that carry reminder advertising messages, and scientific articles, in brochures, in reference books, in package inserts, in digests, and in annotated bibliographies from the scientific literature.

The industry accepts the full responsibility for the promotion of useful knowledge about the drugs they have developed and which have been approved by a governmental bureau. This form of education is a talent that is useful because full understanding is useful; it is not a talent to be hidden under a napkin.

As a physician who has been interested in both teaching and learning, I can attest that our profession benefits from all forms of useful knowledge, since it encourages and stimulates us to apply the best in science to the needs of our patients.

The summation of this glimpse into the function of an industry is that it represents—no, in a larger sense it *is* our national drug supply.

The supply is of little use until it moves out of the industry into the normal channels of distribution.

Often people think of the drug industry in terms of the local pharmacist or the TV commercial for pain relief. Our focus here on this occasion is the prescription drug industry. It has maybe one-thousand manufacturers, and some thirty of these account for most of the production and sales, but in contrast to other industries there are no dominant giants. There are probably ten to fifteen thousand different drug products marketed, but most of the activity takes place with one thousand to fifteen hundred products. In the distribution phase there are three hundred to four hundred wholesale firms that act as depots around the country, and about 53,000 local pharmacies that provide ready availability of needed drugs in every community. Having this immediacy of supply, incidentally, is one of the elements in the cost of prescriptions. Approximately 200,000 physicians are the principal users of these products, either through their office practice or through the nation's eight thousand hospitals.

In these cold statistics are some rather warm problems requiring better understanding. One is a problem of marketing and distribution from the manufacturers to the user. The manufacturers market their product to the physician, who orders it for his patient, who purchases it from the registered pharmacist. This method of distribution is controlled by law, designed to protect the public, and the man who purchases the drug must rely upon and have confidence in his doctor, who is making a choice for his benefit.

THE GREAT FORWARD STEPS OF MEDICINE

The hope has been expressed that at some time in the year 2000 the Lowell Lectures will deal with the subject of the healthy society and not a medicated one.

Sir William Osler was quoted as having said that one of the most serious difficulties with which a doctor has to contend is the desire of man to take medicine, and that it is important to teach patients not to take medicine.

The aim of all medicine is to prevent and cure disease. We have made great strides toward this utopian goal, but we have a long road to travel before we can conquer all disease, illness, and suffering. In Osler's day, or beginning in 1885—when he went to Philadelphia as a clinical professor of medicine and a consultant —there were very few drugs available for the effective treatment of patients and there were no effective drugs for the treatment of most diseases that he and other doctors encountered. In fact there was very little known about most diseases, their causes, their courses, let alone their treatment.

In order to view the contributions of science and industry in therapeutic perspective and to appreciate some of the great forward steps in medicine and the progress in treatment, let us look at the list of drugs that were used by doctors most widely beginning in 1885 down to the present time.

TABLE I

The Ten Most Widely Used Drugs in 1885

Iron chloride for anemia

Quinine for malaria

Ether as anesthesia

Opium and its alkaloids (morphine) for pain

Alcohol as sedative or for pain-relieving effects

Sodium bicarbonate for indigestion

Bromide salts as sedation and for anticonvulsant effects

Mercury and iodides for syphilis

Calomel as a laxative

Paregoric for diarrhea

As you can see, the drugs used at that time by Osler and others were iron for anemia, quinine for malaria, ether as anesthesia, opium and its alkaloids (morphine) for pain, alcohol for its sedative or pain-relieving effects, sodium bicarbonate for indigestion, bromide salts as sedation and for anticonvulsant effects, and mercury and iodides for syphilis. Osler called opium "God's own Medicine," because of its pain-relieving qualities, and from Sydenham's day (1624-1689) down to the present it would be difficult for any doctor to be callous enough to practice medicine without this wonderful pain-relieving remedy.

As we review the situation twenty-five years later, or in 1910, it is a striking fact that in this twenty-five-year period only arsphenamine and antitoxin (diphtheria) had been introduced as great advances in medical therapy. (Digitalis had been known and used occasionally before 1885.) But as knowledge advanced, and research in therapeutics progressed, the list of effective drugs available for the public in 1945 was quite different.

The comparable list could not be made of the ten most widely used drugs, but the ten most widely used *categories* of drugs.

TABLE 2

The Ten Most Widely Used Drugs in 1910

1. Iron
2. Quinine
3. Ether
4. Morphine
5. Alcohol
6. Mercury
7. Iodine
8. Digitalis
9. Diphtheria antitoxin
10. Arsphenamine

They contained insulin, a substance of great significance; the growing roster of antitoxins and vaccines; a new group called vitamins; blood products, including whole blood, plasma, and derivatives. And of course, heading the list is the heart of the medical revolution itself, the anti-infectives—the original miracle drugs, the sulfas, then the super-miracle drug, penicillin.

Finally in the sixties, still another roster, and this time it not only has whole new families of drugs, but no single item can be highlighted. The antibiotics have spread into broad-spectrum and special purpose types; still newer sulfas have taken over; tranquilizers and antidepressants are in our mental hospitals; a whole new era of cardiovascular medicine has been created; steroid chemistry has become a specialty of its own; many diabetics no longer must rely upon injections of insulin to control their disease; newer analgesics have given us greater resources than the salicylates; we have a range of antihistamines for allergic conditions; we have a range of weapons against anemia; the hormone field is undergoing still further transformation with the progestational-estrogenic agents; vitamins continue to supplement our

TABLE 3

The Ten Most Widely Used Categories of Drugs in 1945

Penicillin, sulfonamides,
  other antibiotics
Whole blood, plasma, blood
  derivatives
Quinine, quinacrine
Ether, other anesthetics,
  morphine, cocaine,
  barbiturates
Digitalis
Arsphenamines
Immunizing agents, specific
  antitoxins, vaccines
Insulin, liver extract
Other hormones
Vitamins

nutrition; and we see a procession of polio, influenza, measles, mumps, and other vaccines either in our hands or under development.

THE ANTI-INFECTIVE BREAKTHROUGH

Modern chemotherapy for infectious diseases began with Ehrlich and the introduction of arsphenamine for the treatment of syphilis. Following this great milestone, little progress was made in the discovery of chemicals that were effective in systemic bacterial infections. It was only thirty-two years ago in 1935 that the great breakthrough in the laboratories of Bayer with the discovery by Domagk that azo dye Prontosil had the properties fore-

TABLE 4

The Eleven Most Widely Used Categories of Drugs in the 1960's

Anti-infective agents

Tranquilizing agents

Cardiovascular, diuretic
agents

Steroids

Antidiabetic agents

Analgesics, anesthetics

Antihistamines

Antianemics

Hormones

Vitamins

Biological products

seen by Ehrlich and was capable of curing bacterial infection such as childbed fever, meningitis, and other diseases. This discovery marked the beginning of the present era of bacterial chemotherapy. A few months after this discovery a group of French scientists found that the effect of Prontosil was due to sulfanilamide, which was one of the constituents of Prontosil.

Sulfanilamide is a very simple molecule which can readily be chemically modified. An enormous effort was now made in many industrial research laboratories to obtain derivatives of sulfanilamide with improved properties and different biological activity. Thousands of compounds have been made, and the end is not yet reached. All of the sulfonamides used clinically at the present time came from industrial laboratories, an enormous contribution to human and animal health.

As an extra dividend to the sulfonamide development in the battle against infections, it must be mentioned that at an early stage of their clinical use, it was noticed that some of the products, in particular the urea-substituted sulfonamides, had a blood-sugar-lowering effect similar to that of insulin.

Next, observations by two German pharmaceutical companies led to substances that exhibited the blood-sugar-lowering effect to a pronounced degree. These products and others discovered elsewhere are now used extensively for the treatment of certain mild forms of diabetes, and with remarkable success. They have the advantage that they can be taken by mouth and obviate the necessity of frequent insulin injections. They act to stimulate the production of insulin by the pancreas in cases where the insulin-producing cells are still capable of functioning.

A still further development flowing from the sulfonamides was the discovery of the powerful diuretic action of some members of this class of compound. Once it had been established that sulfanilamide derivatives were capable of removing excessive amounts of salt and water from the body and hence, of potential value in treatment of heart disease, hypertension and some forms of kidney disease, an intensive search was made by industrial laboratories for more effective compounds. Success was achieved and diuretics such as chlorothiazide and others have found widespread and beneficial effects in the diseases where there are disturbances in water and electrolyte metabolism.

Thus the discovery of the sulfonamides was a major triumph for chemotherapy of infections as well as other disorders, but it had a disastrous financial effect on that section of the pharmaceutical industry concerned with the production of antisera against bacterial infections such as pneumonia, where an enormous investment in money, manpower, and research was lost almost overnight. I mention this as one of the typical examples of a professional hazard to which the pharmaceutical industry is exposed.

As the antisera were replaced by the sulfonamides, these were superseded to a large extent by the antibiotics. This meant that many manufacturing companies had to change their research activities and line of business. But it was the beginning of a great period of growth for the industry and for research and advance in therapeutics.

ANTIBIOTICS

The initial observations of the potential power of penicillin made in an academic laboratory did not at once signify that a drug of practical use had become available. The problems of isolation and production in large enough quantities to be of practical use lay ahead, and the research and development that went into the solution of the manufacturing problem was one of the finest examples of cooperative research between industry, government, and academic laboratories that has ever been known in science and industry.

Before penicillin could be produced in sufficient quantities to be available to the public, many new engineering techniques had to be worked out, not only for the fermentation process proper, but also for the large-scale recovery process under sterile conditions. These contributions toward large-scale production of antibiotics came almost exclusively from industry, and they undertook the costly and expensive job with their own resources. The major firms were offered government funds, but did not accept the offer. Rather they accepted the responsibility and risk for developing the product without government aid.

In the entire antibiotic field since penicillin, the industry has not only developed engineering methods for production, but they have discovered or played a key role in developing new antibiotics as well as new and ingenious methods for producing them for clinical use. These include streptomycin, the broad-spectrum antibiotics (tetracyclines), chloramphenicol, and many others.

It should be emphasized that the work on antibiotics, in which our industrial laboratories have played such an important role, has had a dramatic effect on the mortality rate for infectious disease, and most of the severe bacterial infections that were major causes of death and illness thirty years ago can now be effectively controlled. Certainly, in the area of infectious diseases, greater advances have been made in the control of infections through chemotherapy in the last three decades than in the entire previous history of medicine, and our industrial laboratories have played the major role in this advance.

Another area in which our industries have made great advances has been the discovery and production of drugs for the treatment of mental illness, America's number one health problem. While it is generally admitted that many factors have played a part in the advances in care of mentally ill patients, including an increased public interest as well as a demand for improved treatment and an increase in psychiatric personnel, the introduction of "psychiatric" drugs has helped make patients more accessible to treatment, more able to take part in social activities, and has enabled them to carry on in their home or community rather than lead an institutional existence. These radical changes have been felt throughout our society.

The so-called psychopharmacological drugs were developed in our industrial laboratories. The first group, generally known as the tranquilizers, emerged as a by-product of the antihistamine drugs, which are used so widely for the treatment of allergic disorders, such as hay fever and similar conditions. It was noted that some of the effective antihistamines had a sedative effect, and from this observation a systematic attempt was made to modify the structures of these compounds in such a way as to enhance their sedative property. These studies were successful and new compounds were discovered in our industries. These discoveries stimulated the pharmaceutical industries to study a wide variety of chemicals for their effects upon behavior and mental illness. As a result we have available today more and more drugs for the treatment of the mentally ill. The contributions of our industrial laboratories in this area are outstanding, and while they have not replaced other forms of treatment, they have greatly changed them in a positive and beneficial manner.

The contributions of industry to medical therapeutics, as illustrated by the discovery and development of anti-infective agents, can be extended to include the steroids, the newer hormones, oral contraceptive agents, drugs useful in the treatment of high blood pressure, and the biological products used as preventive agents against diseases such as measles, influenza, poliomyelitis.

In enumerating these contributions, I want to make it absolutely clear that the best and most productive results in the field of drug research have flowed from close collaboration between industrial and academic laboratories, and I submit that this collaboration is of the greatest importance for the future.

I shall now leave the technical aspects of my theme and say something about several of the needs, opportunities, and issues of the future.

SOME ISSUES AND OPPORTUNITIES

Looking at this record, we see a quarter-century of progress in drug development—a display linking the industrial, academic, governmental, and professional worlds. Each has contributed, and my thesis is that not the least of these has been the industrial, whose scientific initiative has spurred us forward.

But a question must be asked: Will this quarter-century prove to have been unique? Has either the state-of-the-art or the industrial mechanism itself moved off of the stage and onto the pages of history?

My belief is that they have merely begun to demonstrate their worth: However, their contributions to our health and well-being between now and the year 2000 will be influenced by at least three major debates in public policy, all of which affect patient, physician, and the public. I define these as the issue of professionalism, the issue of economic philosophy, and the issue of national research policy.

These complex themes weave in and out of each other in endless subtle ways.

PROFESSIONALISM

By professionalism I mean principally the status of the private health professions in guiding the health and medical care services of tomorrow. Will these private professions themselves set the standards, or will the general public create standards through governmental legislation and regulations?

That the role of the health professions is being appropriated more and more by public agencies is seen through the entire field of medicine. In drugs, specifically, we are in the midst of a revolution. Since 1938 there has been a progressively greater involvement of government in the control of research, production, sale, and dispensing of drugs. Less and less is the judgment of therapy left to the individual practicing physician. And today the physician might be at some jeopardy if he were to administer an unapproved drug to a patient without registering in advance with the Food and Drug Administration. He might find peril even in using an *approved* drug in a condition for which it has *not* been approved. The sanction of the Federal Food and Drug law, of course, is primarily to bar interstate shipment of drugs if not in compliance with the law, and the physician is seldom engaged in interstate commerce. But his liability in malpractice suits goes up dramatically if his judgment is in conflict with "approved" judgment. The industry supplying him, of course, is indeed vulnerable to governmental prosecution in many ways. It must be careful to tell the physician only those facts or opinions that either have previously been sanctioned by the government or can in no way be labeled as the promotion of useful knowledge. It is no longer up to the physician to assess or evaluate the information supplied to him; rather, his professional jurisdiction has in a sense been restricted to the application of approved knowledge to individual patients.

Using these terms is of course troublesome to me; the phrase "approved knowledge" is alien to the professional and the scientifically trained person. Yet, one cannot reject out of hand the government's desire for consumer protection in matters of health care beyond that given him by his personal physician. Such is reality, and it must be faced.

The problem is whether the new officialism in 1967 will blunt professional judgment and retard advances in therapy that reach beyond those of today.

The import for the drug industry is unclear. You have undoubtedly read of the official adverse criticisms and legal actions (citations, seizures, recommendation for criminal prosecution) taken by the Food and Drug Administration against even some of the most reputable of drug houses on advertising matters in which the agency has judged the companies to be guilty of exaggerations, omissions, or inaccuracies. So often, of course, these are matters of opinion. On how many questions of therapeutic judgment is there a consensus as to detail? I understand fully that the task of carrying out the legislation is difficult indeed and that the agency is trying valiantly to chart a course with few stars for sighting. My plea is that we not write off completely the ability of the doctor of medicine—by dint of his extensive education, training, and experience—to exercise critical judgment on educational material; and that we recognize the legitimate and important role of advocacy in the marketing of drugs. In the still primitive science of medical practice a stamp of official approval may itself prove misleading, and lull the practitioner into a false sense of security as he forgets that *behind* the seal of government approval also lies human judgment, sincere though it may be.

ECONOMIC PHILOSOPHY

The second issue is that of economic philosophy. Although my training and experience may qualify me to speak of medical judgments and research policy, they do not equip me as an economist. Let me allude to this vastly interesting subject, however, lest you think I fail to recognize a highly sensitive public issue.

With the mounting costs of medical care, the price of different services (hospital, professional, nursing, insurance, and administrative) has been subject to vigorous discussion, investigation, and debate, and this applies to drugs and medical supplies. Various issues concerning medical care costs have been raised by the public, as government programs have become increasingly involved in financing these costs, again including the price of drugs.

The price structure of any article as well as any service is an extremely complex matter; highly technical considerations must obviously play a predominant part and this applies naturally to drugs and medicine. To claim that this or that drug is expensive has little or no meaning; the question is, expensive in relation to what? To its quality, to the total cost of medical care, to its total developmental production and distribution cost, to the purchasing power of the buyer and user, to the value of its effect, or to the level of its profit?

It is impossible for the ordinary citizen and the consumer to assess the price structure of any drug, just as it is impossible for a nontechnologist to express a sound opinion on the price of a battleship, an airplane, a motor car, an electric typewriter, or an atomic bomb.

From what has been said about the contributions of the drug industry, it is important for all of us to understand that the process of discovering, developing, producing, and distributing drugs is time-consuming and expensive and one must take into account the many failures, the professional hazards, the rapid obsolescence, and the frequent replacement of one good drug with a better one, and therefore its limited lifetime as a commercially profitable article must be taken into account. Other factors that need to be understood are the educational and professional service costs. It is the responsibility of the drug manufacturers to inform the doctor, and through him the patient, about the therapeutic usefulness of the drugs that are prescribed. It is the physician's responsibility, and one that he accepts, to decide whether he will prescribe a given medicine for his patient. He makes the decision based upon the facts and evidence presented to him through many media, and the needs of his patient. To aid in the promotion of useful knowledge, the manufacturer uses the mass media. This includes all educational and professional sources, reminder advertising in medical journals written for physicians, brochures, annotated bibliographies, package inserts, all mailing pieces describing a medicine, all films, slides, charts and published monographs, scientific and commercial exhibits at medical meetings, and visits by professional service personnel to physicians. All of these sources and educational aids cost money, but they are necessary and essential expenses and must be added to the total cost of a product.

What I am stressing here is that in our present system of competitive research, production, and marketing, the over-all cost of drugs to the people who require them needs to be related to many factors. It is a highly specialized field and one for the experts in economics. The ordinary citizen as well as the members of the health professions recognize the public issue of medical care economics, of which drug prices are only one element. What we need to understand is that our drug manufacturers are striving to produce new drugs for people at a price they can afford to pay and make them available to all who need them as a part of their health care. They are not just duplicating products of known material; they are encouraging new trends in therapy through the development of new drugs and promoting their use to the professions who take care of the sick.

NATIONAL RESEARCH POLICY

At the present time and extending into the future, the problem of a national research policy with respect to medicine and drugs is being examined in great detail. The harmonious collaboration between industrial, governmental, and academic scientists and institutions in the area of biomedical research holds great promise for future therapeutics. But today's biochemical research efforts and the ultimate application of new knowledge raise the important question of how these research sources will be managed and directed in the years ahead. Definite objectives and priorities are being established by scientists, experts in management and administration, statesmen, politicians, and the general public.

In the development of a future national research policy it will be essential to define the boundaries and divisions of responsibility between governmental, academic, and industrial groups. Each has special abilities, and it is highly important to identify the areas and the tasks that each group can do best. There are many tasks that academic and governmental laboratories can do, which industrial laboratories can't do. There are many tasks that industrial laboratories can do well when they stick to what they know best and have the strongest incentives for accomplishment. Experience has shown that under our present system government does well when it works in harmony rather than at cross purposes with the dynamic forces of research in industry and academia. Certainly the academic community and government-supported laboratories are in the best position to make their greatest contributions in breaking new ground and searching for a better understanding of the fundamental laws of nature. Priorities must be given the intellectual investment in this type of inquiry.

Yet the public is impatient and in a hurry for new drugs to fight disease. Our privately supported research establishments, as well as our industrial laboratories, have set as their highest priority not only the development of new knowledge, but its application, and they do this in the shortest period of time between discovery and application. The private performance as measured against both research opportunity and the public interest indicates that our industries are prepared to concentrate their efforts and expend their money and other resources on the developmental aspects of research; that is, what they do best and most efficiently.

Past experience has demonstrated that a diverse program of research support and direction is needed to achieve the best results. Functions should not overlap, and no group should gain advantage over the other. Relationships need to be improved; academic centers, voluntary health associations, medical societies, private foundations, and industry need to be encouraged to take their own approaches to the difficult decisions of research planning and evaluation. Science thrives best when it has maximum options of support and interests, and operates in a climate and environment of creativity.

Industry's research productivity, primarily self-financed, has demonstrated over the past thirty years its ability to produce— which is a sign of greatness, and a sign of private competence and initiative.

Our research establishments will make their greatest contribution to the physician, the patient, and the public if they plan jointly and recognize the opportunity for advance through establishing priorities for various groups and developing a policy in which diverse support of research is recognized.

We need to guard against a monolithic, centrally controlled and directed national research policy, which would impede, interfere with, or prevent the effective discovery of new drugs and their development for the public.

I hope that I have made it quite clear that I consider modern drugs to be one of the greatest blessings of our time. Notwithstanding the important contributions to the promotion of health by our scientists in universities and research institutions, our hospitals, our practitioners of medicine and nursing, and the other members of the health professions, the discovery, development, production, and availability of new drugs without the active and energetic participation of the pharmaceutical industry would be impossible.

The future is bright for continuing advance in the area of health improvement, including the contributions that can be made by industry providing all groups in our society—academic, governmental, and industrial—define their roles and work together in a spirit of hearty and harmonious collaboration.

NOTE ON CONTRIBUTOR

Chester S. Keefer is consultant to the dean of Boston University School of Medicine and Wade Professor Emeritus, Boston University, Boston, Massachusetts. He was graduated from Bucknell University (B.S. 1918, M.S. 1922) and Johns Hopkins University School of Medicine, 1922. He is a past president of the American College of Physicians and of the American Clinical and Climatological Association. In honor of his wartime efforts directing the civil distribution of penicillin, streptomycin, and cortisone, he was honored by both the United States and Great Britain. During World War II he also served on the Surgeon General's commission on hemolytic streptococcus infections and as a consultant to the Secretary of War. He has also been a special assistant for health and medical affairs to the United States Department of Health Education and Welfare and was consultant on the development of standards of the Kerr-Mills legislation for that department in 1960. He has authored many books and pamphlets on medicine, infectious diseases, and medical education.

12

The Role of Government

JAMES L. GODDARD, M.D.

My PRESENTATION IS supposed to be "the last word" on the subject of this fascinating series, *The Medicated Society*. Let me hastily note two things: *First,* the problems surrounding the advancement of health in our society are too complex for a last word. I believe all previous lecturers in this series have left you with that impression, also. *Second,* I doubt that a government administrator should be regarded as a final or absolute authority.

Please make no mistake. I am truly honored to have an opportunity to present a view of the government's role—past, present, and possibly future—in the development of a better living environment and the maintenance of some rational control over medication in our society.

But good government is not just responsible—it is responsive. It is given assignments by the governed. As government officials we may carry out these responses with imagination, economy, verve, dedication, and occasionally brilliance. The illusion may be that the entire process—from the discovery of the problem to its ultimate, breathtaking solution—is totally the work of government. But that is usually not the case.

At this point, then, let us assume that there is yet one more presentation to be made. The one that goes beyond the views of the professionals, the scientists, the administrators—that is, if you will, a synergism of what you have thus far. It is the presentation that each of you will, for himself, put together as a reasonable "last word" in this series.

It has been my pleasure to review several of the prior presentations. My hosts in the Lowell lecture series have been attentive to this matter, and I hope, therefore, that I can repay them—and you—with some material that may be new and will fill out in a useful way the panorama described thus far.

I want very much to begin with a rational view of a major issue. Yet, while browsing through some historical materials in preparation for this discussion, I was struck with the difficulty of always finding reason and of being able to cling to it with full assurance. What are the great truths to begin with? And, among them, where does our problem of health care fit?

Here's a great truth written by Grover Cleveland in the April 1905 issue of *The Ladies' Home Journal:* "Sensible and responsible women do not want to vote," wrote the ex-President. "The relative positions to be assumed by man and woman in the working out of our civilization were assigned long ago by a higher intelligence than ours."

1905 was one of those years, I imagine, even for the *Journal.* In another article, the magazine did an exposé of certain patent medicines. It singled out Mrs. Winslow's Soothing Syrup as a great danger. The syrup was used to quiet down teething babies. But it contained morphine. The British wouldn't allow it to be sold in the Isles without the word "poison" printed on the label. That was rather shocking to a number of *Journal* readers.

That was also the year the United States Supreme Court ruled that a State could enact and enforce a compulsory vaccination law. The case was *Jacobson vs. Massachusetts* and Massachusetts—and the nation—won a major health victory.

It was a yeasty time in our history. Values were under review. In the following year, 1906, President Theodore Roosevelt spoke to the Gridiron Club in Washington and mentioned the "muckrakers," which seems to have been the first time the word was used in its modern sense. The President was referring to writers like Ida Tarbell, David Graham Phillips, Lincoln Steffens, and of course Upton Sinclair.

Sinclair's book, *The Jungle,* had tremendous impact on America, and the shock waves reached deep into Washington, as President Roosevelt was aware. *The Jungle* focused principally on the meat-packing industry and helped bring about passage of the Meat Packing Act of 1906. The day Congress passed the Meat Packing Act—that was June 30, 1906—it also passed the Federal Food and Drugs Act of 1906.

If Sinclair was a "muckraker" *outside* the government, I suppose you could say that Dr. Harvey Washington Wiley was a kind of "muckraker" *inside* the government. He had been chief of the Bureau of Chemistry in the Department of Agriculture since 1883 and agitated for twenty-three years until the Federal Food and Drugs Law was passed.

There was little doubt that the law was needed. The teething syrup was a minor example. Boric acid was widely used as a commercial food preservative at the time, but it was hardly to be mentioned on a package label. Butter was sold as butter, even though it was heavily laced with other fats, including lard. Basically, the law was passed to prevent such adulterations. For example, ten days before the law was passed, James Mann told the Congress of the kinds of things found in everyday supplies of coffee. It was "colored with Scheele's green, iron oxide, yellow ochre, chrome yellow, burnt umber, Venetian red, tumeric, Prussian blue, and indigo; adulterated with roasted peas, beans, wheat, rye, oats, chicory, brown bread, charcoal, red slate, bark, and date stones."

Dr. Wiley and his volunteer "poison squad" received the enforcement authority they had so patiently and valiantly sought.

The tiny Bureau of Chemistry, with less than fifty people, took on the job of carrying out the first Act from which a number of laws have since sprung and from which today's Food and Drug

Administration itself—with nearly five thousand employees—has itself grown.

Among the opposers of the Federal Food and Drugs Law were the manufacturers, distributors, and retailers of foods and drugs. This is formidable opposition. And I use the present tense, by the way. But I would like to quote from a little publication produced in August 1911. It was called "Kellogg's *Square Dealer,* a Monthly Message of Good Cheer from the Home of 'The Sweetheart of the Corn.' "

Dr. Wiley had by then spent five hectic years as chief food inspector for the United States. He was not easily intimidated. That is why, the *Square Dealer* reported to its forty thousand readers, "They are after Wiley's scalp in Washington right now. It has been recommended, with the Attorney General's endorsement, that he be 'permitted to resign for the good of the service.' " The *Square Dealer* admitted that "Dr. Wiley has made mistakes like the rest of us. He has had ample opportunity, for he has been *doing things.* The only man who doesn't make mistakes is the man who is loafing on the job." But Kellogg's went right down the line for Dr. Wiley, even drafting a sample form letter for food distributors to use to write President Taft. The letter read, "I believe Dr. Harvey W. Wiley, chief of the Bureau of Chemistry, to be an honest, fearless and efficient official, the loss of whose services would be a calamity to the country. I respectfully protest against his proposed dismissal."

The magazine explained its position even more clearly. "We who are in the business of making and distributing foods realize best how much vigilance is required to weed out the humbuggery, the quackery, the rank dishonesty that would otherwise fasten its blood-sucking tentacles upon this business."

Now this was the voice of Kellogg—Dr. John Harvey Kellogg, who firmly believed that special food combinations could do more for you than any dozen doctors. And it was to Dr. Kellogg's sanitarium in Battle Creek that Upton Sinclair went for the cure

—the cure consisting of the most artful filling and evacuation of the stomach and bowel then known to contemporary man.

Thus, Dr. Wiley—the so-called "Father of the Federal Food and Drugs Act"—had some unpredictable allies. Less than a year after Dr. Kellogg's *Square Dealer* so loudly endorsed him, Dr. Wiley resigned.

With the exception of the passage of the Sherley Amendment in 1912—the year of Harvey Wiley's new freedom—most enforcement activity for more than three decades centered upon foods. And the Sherley Amendment was a kind of footnote, passed to prohibit the labeling of medicines with false and fraudulent therapeutic claims.

But there was evidence building up that the public needed broader protection. In January 1933, *100,000,000 Guinea Pigs* by F. J. Schlink, revealed the horrors in the marketplace. By the time Franklin Delano Roosevelt was inaugurated as our thirty-second President, the book had gone through several editions. During President Roosevelt's famous Hundred Days, Assistant Secretary of Agriculture Rexford Guy Tugwell drew up a new bill to expand dramatically the government's role in foods, drugs, and cosmetics.

"The Tugwell Bill" had a stormy career. Everyone was against it, except for Schlink and Arthur Kallet and J. B. Matthews, and an array of new consumer protection groups. There was also a handful of legislators and government administrators who, together, finally put through the Federal Food, Drug, and Cosmetic Act of 1938.

The Federal Food, Drug, and Cosmetic Act is the basic statute under which the Food and Drug Administration exercises its jurisdiction over drugs and devices. Its main contributions were the requirements that all new drugs coming into the marketplace after 1938 first had to be proved safe by the manufacturer and be more carefully labeled.

The hard, new accent on drug safety was a reflection of the "Elixir of Sulfanilamide" disaster. Sulfanilamide was a "miracle drug." Everyone was reading about it in the newspapers of the late 1930's. A small entrepreneur mixed sulfanilamide with diethylene glycol, found that it looked and tasted all right, and began selling it. Very soon, the concoction took 107 lives, most of them children.

The "new drug" provisions of the FDC Act, therefore, were passed in the aftermath of the Elixir of Sulfanilamide episode, when drug safety was a real issue of the day. Later Amendments to the Act were variations on this theme. The Durham-Humphrey Amendment established the difference between prescription and nonprescription drugs. Prescription drugs were those that could not be used safely without medical supervision. The Color Additive Amendments of 1960 gave the FDA the power to set safe limits for colors used in drugs, as well as in foods and cosmetics.

Then the Kefauver-Harris Amendments of 1962 went beyond safety to the issues of effectiveness and reliability: Does the drug do what its label says it will do? Once again, after years of hearings and formidable opposition by industry and even many segments of the medical profession, the new, stronger law was passed. It passed Congress unanimously in October 1962—three months after The Washington *Post* revealed the story of thalidomide and how an FDA medical officer, Dr. Frances O. Kelsey, had kept the European drug out of the United States under the slim regulations of the old 1938 law. Thousands of babies had been born malformed in Europe because their mothers took the seemingly mild antinausea drug during pregnancy. But the full machinery of government was not available to protect American mothers and babies until the tragedy of the thalidomide deaths and the passage of the Kefauver-Harris Amendments.

This machinery is, therefore, relatively new and there has been —and will continue to be—a great deal of discussion interpretation, misinterpretation, and even litigation on the expanded law and regulations set out by the Food and Drug Administration. I don't believe we have the luxury of time that prior generations have had to work out differences of opinion on all points. I think this very series illustrates that fact. We need to know a great deal right now, and we must have a great deal of assurance that what we know is up-to-date and correct. Therefore, under our present law a massive collection of data must be marshaled into proper form and perspective before a drug can be put into general use in our society.

Basically, the Federal Food, Drug, and Cosmetic Act, as amended, requires that manufacturers do more than merely submit safety data—data that show the drug as not being harmful. Today the distribution and use of drugs during their investigational stages is controlled by law. The information from these investigational trials must prove that the drug is effective—as well as safe—for the intended use or uses. And the law also requires that the advertising and promotion of approved drugs must be carried out so that the prescribing physician, the nurse, the pharmacist, or whoever actually does carry out the drug therapy will have full knowledge of the effects of the drug, the good as well as the bad—indications and contraindications, side effects, precautions, warnings, and anything else that shows a balanced view of the drug's potential.

I must say that all three of these basic components of our drug law have come under heavy attack since 1962, yet they stand up quite well. The provision surrounding the investigational uses of new drugs have been broadly criticized by professionals in industry and medicine. Because the government has required that the investigator actually file an investigational plan, that he have some rational approach to his experimentations on human patients, that he be able to put his facts together in some understandable way, and that his subjects or those responsible for them know what is going on—because of these requirements, some critics have charged the government with curtailing investigations and discouraging good people from entering the investigational new drug field.

Frankly, I see no sharp downward curve in the number of clinical investigators working with new drugs. We have about

25,000 investigators on file. I see no drop in the literature on new drugs. On the contrary, it appears that investigational work has been made, if anything, a good deal more professional and with more actual protection for the investigator than was previously the case. Certainly the sponsors of investigations—the drug manufacturers, chiefly—have benefited to a large extent because a degree of order and responsibility has now been imposed where only a minimum existed before. It is a bit easier to look ahead at the payoff from a new drug, once you know what the legal and budgetary requirements are going to look like during the term of the proposed investigational trials.

The Congress said that there must be "substantial evidence" that a drug will be effective for its claimed uses, or as the law itself reads, "that the drug will have the effect it purports or is represented to have under the conditions of use prescribed, recommended, or suggested in the labeling or proposed labeling thereof."

This is, of course, an area of controversy regarding every new single entity or compound. Efficacy can be quite relative, unless there is good and reasonably lengthy clinical experience with the drug during the investigational stage.

But again, should the government maintain an oppressive hold on approvals, letting the drugs appear infrequently and only after seemingly interminable investigational trials? Or should the government allow the marketplace to be the final arbiter, allowing sales to be the true barometer of drugs approved after minimal testing? These alternatives are the extremes, of course, but they are still gallantly expressed by some of our leaders in medicine and business. Fortunately, there is a broad space in the center where the rest of us can join together and move forward with the investigational and approval processes with some degree of professional pride, respect, and real accomplishment regarding drug efficacy.

I mentioned that the FDC Act included provisions that covered "all advertisements and other descriptive printed matter issued or caused to be issued by the manufacturer, packer, or distributor," and so forth. This third major component of the 1962 amendments has been the subject of debate over the past year. There have been some unfortunate abuses, some innocent misunderstandings, and some old-fashioned Indian wrestling— tests of strength between government and private industry.

The law is clear enough. So are the regulations. But such statements are again too simplistic to handle the range of "descriptive printed matter" on which Congress asked us to keep tabs.

We review medical journal advertising and convention exhibits.

We screen films and filmstrips.

We listen to recordings.

We see slides.

We read direct mail.

We give our own presentations.

We go to hearings, and we even go to court.

It is a complicated business because the subject matter— chemotheraphy—is itself complex and because the full range of media is being employed by those who market FDA-approved drugs.

We are not going to turn back the clock on either the drugs or the media. Nor should we at this point lay on an oppressive hand because—let us please admit—it is through advertising that most busy physicians get their messages about drugs. So it is entirely possible that the government's role, if too assiduously followed, could in fact restrict the ability of the health professional to know what he had to know about drugs in order to prescribe and administer them properly.

Let me repeat a statement made earlier: The government responds to the needs of the public. In the matter of drug therapy, the government has thus far moved forward into those areas where real public protection was needed. The legislative histories behind the major acts and amendments are lengthy and impressive. The shock of an Elixir of Sulfanilamide or a thalidomide episode has been a final demonstration of need that has usually been prescribed by years of other evidence and testimony.

Fortunately, legislative hearings culminating in some human tragedy may no longer be the pattern of relief. We may be arriving at a more rational plateau upon which we may order our society and its medical care. For example, I am reminded of *The Rockefeller Panel Reports,* which were published during the late 1950's. They were collected and published in 1961 under the title, *Prospect for America.* Among the thirty-three distinguished panelists who drew together the ideas and at that time "prospects" were Lucius Clay, John Gardner, Oveta Culp Hobby, James Killian, the late Henry Luce, Charles Percy, Jacob Potofsky, Dean Rusk, and Edward Teller.

"Health," said the panelists, "in its broadest aspects has an importance to our Nation second only to our National security." Turning to "Medical Research," they concluded:

The toll of today's leading killing and crippling diseases, such as cancer, cardiovascular diseases, and mental illness, is staggering in both human and economic terms. In addition, many new types of health problems and opportunities are emerging today that demand intensive investigation.

The acquisition of new knowledge is basic to advancing national health. We recommend, therefore, continued expansion of our medical research programs as rapidly as the supply of scientific talent will permit.

As we step up medical research efforts, equal strides must be taken toward putting these results to use more rapidly. We recommend that public health authorities and private medical groups join in a study analyzing the extent of the time lag between the acquisition of new medical knowledge and its practical availability to the general public, identifying the causes of delay and delineating measures to reduce it.

The report goes on to speak of "Medical Manpower" and points to a possible decline in the ratio of doctors to total population. That decline is, in fact, taking place right now. The report also called for increased training of professional and practical nurses.

As for "Medical Facilities," the panelists noted that "the increase in chronic disease and the needs of an aging population highlight the necessity for substantial expansion of facilities for long-term care, particularly high quality nursing homes for the care of the aged with moderate impairments." There was a call for "developing radically new types of medical facilities, such as hospitals permitting maximum self-help and community care centers offering diagnostic services and extensive outpatient treatment and homemaker services."

As to the subject of costs, *The Rockefeller Panel Report* came out for group medical practice "with essentially all costs prepaid by the subscribers through family health insurance premiums." In addition, the panelists "urge as a major objective of prepayment plans over the next decade the coverage of doctor's and nursing care *outside* the hospital. Such coverage can serve as a real encouragement to early discovery and treatment of physical defects and illness, thereby resulting in better health and lower costs, and to shorter periods of hospitalization."

I have possibly been too lean in my excerpts, but I do want you to grasp the major areas of concern of the section on "Health and Medical Care." They were pulled together between 1958 and 1960 and published in book form in 1961.

Since that time the government has responded in a number of vital ways. The Executive and the Legislative branches have put into effect a number of programs that these private citizens projected as vital to our Nation—"second only to our National security." These measures include:

Medicare—Health Insurance for the Aged
Regional Medical Programs Act for Heart Disease, Cancer, and Stroke
The Nurse Training Act
Manpower Development and Training Amendments for Health Service Occupations

The Older Americans Act

The Maternal and Child Health and Mental Retardation Planning Amendments to the Social Security Act

Community Mental Health Centers Act

Vocational Rehabilitation Amendments for Innovation Projects

Public Works and Economic Development Act

Hill-Burton Act Amendments for Urban Facilities Improvement

Children's Immunization Act

Many other vital pieces of legislation have been enacted by the Congress and signed by the President to enlarge our capacity to care for all our citizens—regardless of race or geographical location.

In this year's Message to the Congress on Health and Education, President Johnson laid out four basic aims:

To expand our knowledge of disease and our research and development of better ways to deliver health care to every American;

To build our health resources, by stepped-up training of health workers and by improved planning of health facilities;

To remove barriers to good medical care for those who most need care;

To strengthen our partnership for health by encouraging regional, state, and local efforts—public and private—to develop comprehensive programs serving all our citizens.

A vast and obvious change in attitude now prevails in this country regarding health protection, although only a scant sixty years have gone by since the passage of the original Federal Food and Drugs Act. Greater initiative is now expected by the governed from government, even though the guides for action—the general directions in which government should move—are still drawn from many expressions of need. While our way of life today may be infinitely more complex, we are more rational about solving each problem as we isolate it.

There has been, then, a balancing off in the course of the past six decades. And we would hope this balance can be maintained in the future as well. But within that broad view of health care we can identify a few details that deserve careful attention. Naturally, the details that catch my attention are also close to the subject of these lectures: medication, drug therapy, the new "chemistry of humankindness."

Today, the pharmaceutical industry is quite deep in research—over a million dollars a day, according to their leading association's own figure. Such vast sums are not spent idly, although to be quite frank, the way these figures are derived is not always clear.

But in amongst the numbers one can identify the effects of the present and the hints of the future. We see extensive activity in drugs affecting the central nervous system. Pediatric dosages of these and other kinds of drugs—antibiotics and antispasmodics, for example—are coming along, as new attention is swinging to infant and child health services. For the other end of the age scale we see more activity in the cardiovascular field, including the anticoagulants and vasodilators. There are the diuretics and the corticosteroids as well. And the new conception control agents have been moving through the current new-drug procedures and finding their role in group comprehensive care units, as well as in private practice.

These are prescription drugs. But nonprescription drugs are also moving along with the same strength: cough and cold preparations, pain relievers, antacids, balms, salves, dressings, and ointments. And there are more on the way.

Ahead of us is an era of drug development and marketing that is surely to be as fascinating as the past era has been, from a purely biomedical viewpoint: anticancer agents, antiarthritics, drugs that alter the genetic code, menopausal drugs, more psychopharmacologicals, synthetic hormones, radiopharmaceuticals, immunochemistry, aging chemotherapy. The list is long.

Let us return, then, to the basic question posed here: What is the role of the government in a medicated society? The premise is clear enough: that society will continue to benefit—"benefit" seems the most appropriate term to use—from drug research, development, and marketing. However, these benefits can be assured to the public only if agencies that are responsible wholly to the public are monitoring this drug activity. The more sophisticated the development of new drugs, the more sophisticated will be this monitoring function by government. Again we will respond to a clear public need, and we will not wait for thalidomide episodes to impress us with our responsibilities.

In addition there is a task that is even more complicated, but in many ways just as important as monitoring the flow of new drugs into the new channels of medical practice. I am speaking of the total surveillance task. We have a need—right now, today—to retrieve better data on the actions and interactions of today's vast supply of drugs, some seven thousand of them. Medical science is a long way from having a good data collection system. In addition we need to know a great deal more about the actions and interactions of drugs with other kinds of chemicals in our environment: additives in our foods or pollutants in our water and air, for example.

Once again we know that this kind of information is vital for science to move ahead on a rational basis. We know that this kind of information is vital for all of society to move ahead on a rational basis.

I am reminded of the statement by Archimedes: "Give me a place to stand and I will move the universe." That place to stand cannot be a random spot of ground. It cannot be cluttered with the rubbish of poor science or commercial speculation. On such terms, the universe will not be moved.

We may know the chemistry—but we must also know the man.

We may know the power—but we must also know control.

We *can* stand for values that have proved sound, for procedures that have proved reasonable and profitable, and for responses to public need that have proved effective.

If we are going to continue our commitment to protecting the lives of all our citizens through expanded health services, then we are indeed going to be a society well outfitted with a variety of old and new medications. Rather than fear the prospect, rather than deny the role of balance and control, I—and I'm sure many of you, also—welcome the challenge of the future and may even be somewhat eager to see if we, as citizens and as human beings, can find our spot on the frontier of health, stand firm, and indeed move the universe.

NOTE ON CONTRIBUTOR

James L. Goddard (M.D., 1949, George Washington School of Medicine, Washington, D.C.) is former commissioner of the Food and Drug Administration and assistant surgeon-general of the Public Health Service of the United States Department of Health, Education and Welfare. He holds a Master's degree in Public Health from Harvard University School of Public Health in 1955. He has served as chief of the Communicable Disease Center of the Public Health Service in Atlanta, Georgia, 1962-1966; and chief of the Accident Prevention Program (PHS-HEW) 1956-1959; and was Civil Air Surgeon for the Federal Aviation Agency from 1959-1962.

Commentary

SAMUEL PROGER, M.D.

THE THOUGHTFUL VIEWS presented in this series of Lowell Lectures on "The Medicated Society" record far more than the present, portentous state of drug use; they log the Protean trip of the past through the ages of drug discovery.

It is an amazing journey, one that has brought physicians and patients of today to an unprecedented, wonderful-terrible point in time where the boundaries between drug use and misuse grow ever more shadowy, while the alternate possibilities for medical good or social evil become truly awesome.

The lectures in a sense comprise a pause in this pilgrimage, a moment taken for reflection and an important, clarifying look at the current kaleidoscope of medicines and diseases and the interplay now recognized between the two. The lecturers have cited the twentieth century benchmarks of advance, pharmaceutical advantages now secured: the extensive degree of infection control by antibiotics; life-sustaining gains wrought by agents against heart and blood vessel diseases; the crucial foot-in-the-door beginning that has come with chemical compounds to modify mental disorders; some measure, though certainly not enough, of chemotherapeutic control over certain forms of cancer; the importance of the first foolproof oral contraceptive; the burgeoning of disease-preventive vaccines and the welcome advent of better palliatives against pain. But the benefits have come at the price of new problems or a multiplication of old ones: drug-induced diseases, perilous side-effects and monstrous fetal insult. The authorities readily admit, too, the limitations still hampering physicians—the absence of curative drugs for the formidable array of crippling, if not killing, chronic degenerative diseases, to name but one vast area of difficulty.

Moreover, the lecturers, sensitive to the worrisome new role being assigned to drugs by laymen, point to the growing dependence on drugs, not for health but for social-psychological reasons. They discuss the rediscovery by modern man of the hallucinogens, the so-called mind-expanders, which primitive people knew in natural forms and used for quasireligious experiences. Today, however, the substances are regarded as ingestable tickets for a new kind of "trip"; escape not only from daily pressure but a ride right out of this world into a no man's land, gambling that it be a heaven, but chancing a hell. Others today would have drugs replace any form of self-discipline be it moderation in eating or drinking or even the mastering of moodiness.

And finally the lecturers have presented their case, as it must be, against a backdrop of ethical considerations, problems intensified by the rush of new drug discovery, and within the framework of regulations and mechanisms for control to assure purity and efficacy.

From his eminent position in the field of clinical pharmacology, Dr. Lasagna has given us a panoramic view of some of the great peaks in the history of drugs. Of help in comprehending this broad expanse is his sorting out of certain *leitmotifs,* or dominant and recurring themes.

He urges that folk remedies not be forgotten or neglected since they represent a rich and still-to-be-mined source of drugs.

It is well established what can and has been accomplished by the talented individual with genius, with good fortune, and with what Pasteur called the "prepared mind."

There is no denying the impetus provided by the opportunity for profit, and he has spelled out both the advantages and disavantages inherent in this drive.

Regarding social control, he demonstrated the need for a balanced approach, one that steers a path between no control and too much control, between freedom to introduce too many drugs and the inability to introduce enough safe, effective and, possibly, even lifesaving drugs. Clearly the aim should be to establish controls that provide the optimal ratio of drug efficacy to drug safety.

The final *motif* is what he calls "the clinical point-counterpoint between uncontrolled chance observations and rigorous experimentation." Both approaches have yielded advances in the past and promise to be productive in the future. Today, however, the rigorously controlled experimental approach is in the ascendancy, since it decreases the number of risky and worthless drugs and increases the number that are reliable and useful.

Dr. Lasagna cautions against smugness with reference to our accomplishments. We are said to be in a golden age, he observes, but notes that there still are vast areas of ignorance. While these are not so vast as they were years ago, it is of interest to remember that Osler in an essay in the 1890's referred to that period as *the golden age of medicine*. Indeed it was a golden age, what with such noteworthy advances as anesthesia and antisepsis, the flowering of bacteriology, and the development of major public health measures for the control of infectious, particularly communicable, diseases. But Osler could do little or nothing for patients with diabetes, pernicious anemia, pneumonia, meningitis, and a host of other diseases. On the other hand, today medicine can do comparatively little, as Dr. Lasagna points out, for most of the degenerative diseases, most cancers, the whole group of noninfectious inflammatory diseases, such as rheumatoid arthritis, ulcerative colitis, and the so-called collagen diseases. In truth, we still have large dark areas. We still have a sound basis for humility, for much of what we think we know is uncertain and most of what we need to know is unknown.

In another area, new lights are being illumined. But the flashing mosaic of previously unexplored pathways of insight for the psychedelic kickster may blind more than it illuminates.

Nevertheless, of the best known of the hallucinogenic drugs, LSD, Dr. Louria says, clinically it "may be potentially beneficial." He lists the areas of potential benefit as follows: chronic alcoholism; sexual abnormalities; schizophrenic children; psychoneurosis; psychopaths; and terminal disease. But how potentially beneficial is it, in fact, for he goes on to say of alcoholism that "studies are not entirely convincing"; of sexual abnormalities that "data are currently far too meager"; of schizophrenia that the drug "may effect improvement" and of psychopaths that "the data are clearly insufficient." It appears that the benefits are not *proved* in any of the conditions he named.

Nonetheless, with respect to the psychoneuroses and terminal illnesses, LSD apparently does show real promise. As to terminal disease, there is no disputing that anything that might provide what he calls "equanimity in the face of imminent death" is worthwhile. But in regard to the psychoneuroses, it is important to recognize the enormous influence of suggestion on the symptoms of a psychoneurosis. The factor of suggestibility is noted with the use of any new drug, and especially one known to have powerful effects. Placebos, for example, will relieve many symptoms in many patients with neuroses: a patient's report of improvement, therefore, is not the same as a good pharmacological effect.

It is reasonable only to say at this point that with certain specific exceptions such as terminal illness we already know enough about LSD to hold that the possible therapeutic benefits are far outweighed by the actual as well as potential hazards. Generally speaking, there is no justification for using a drug in which the ratio of benefit to risk is so low as with LSD. For this is indeed a low-benefit, high-risk drug.

The chief value of LSD, therefore, may be, as Dr. Louria suggests, in its use as a tool to study emotional reactions; to learn something about the effect of certain chemicals on the psyche, with the hope that we may ultimately be able to manipulate drugs to the benefit of the psyche.

As for marihuana, Dr. Louria finds that the moderate use of less potent preparations is generally harmless. He lists, however, a few apparently valid conclusions, some of which are cause for real concern:

1. It can produce acute panic reactions.

2. The more potent cannabis preparations may be associated with criminality.

3. Marihuana, if used chronically (more than ten cigarettes daily), may induce a psychosis.

4. It may make a person more accident prone.

5. It does not lead to the use of addicting drugs.

6. It causes neither addiction nor physical deterioration.

Marihuana, then, has a much better ratio of benefit to harm than LSD, and hence raises different questions. These questions deal with such intangible and ill-defined areas as personal freedom, social pressures, and moral concepts. Just what are the social, legal, emotional, and medical boundaries that we must establish? Is hedonism indeed an unjustifiable basis for drug usage? No one questions the propriety of using drugs to cure or to minimize the effects of illness and to relieve troublesome or annoying symptoms. The same apparently may be said of drugs to ease unhappy responses to life's stresses. We need only note the tremendous consumption of sedatives or so-called tranquilizers. These drugs seem to help some people: They certainly are not harmless. But the question now confronting us is: May drugs also be used just to add a feeling of well being or a sense of pleasure, that is for hedonistic purposes? In a sense we now use drugs in uncontrolled fashion for such purposes, namely caffein (coffee), nicotine (cigarettes), and alcohol. The principal arguments against the use of marihuana for similar purposes have been presented by Dr. Louria. Are they sufficient? He speaks of the incongruity of adding a large number of marihuana inebriates to the already large number of persons inebriated by alcohol. Obviously this would be bad. We may perhaps have the opportunity to prevent the development of a large-scale marihuana problem. Speculatively, the question might well be asked, what might we do if the situation with marihuana and alcohol were reversed; if we were faced with the problem of preventing the abuses of alcohol before its use became widespread. The same question applies to ordinary cigarette smoking.

To repeat, is hedonism or a positive sense of pleasure, really an unjustifiable basis for drug usage? There are many who would gladly exchange a feeling of well-being for the slight risk that a drug like marihuana might entail. This is not to be interpreted as condoning its use. Rather, the question is raised only to indicate that, while the approach to the LSD problem seems fairly clear and reasonable, the same cannot be said of marihuana. Indeed, as Dr. Louria has said, we do need "a total revamping of our narcotic-hallucinogen laws," tightening some and perhaps loosening others.

The basis upon which to make individual and social decisions and all others derives, of course, from man's singular ability to acquire and transmit knowledge from one member of society to another.

Though it may seem far-fetched at first, this leads directly to a far larger problem, the teeming numbers of people who now are threatening to overpopulate the world. In the chapter dealing with global control of population Dr. Rock states that the human species has been perpetuated so far within the structure of monogamous marriage. This would appear to be a simple statement of fact. What is not so simple or obvious is the interesting concept that he offers to the effect that "to ensure perpetuation of the species, parents must have knowledge and must make certain of its transmission to their offspring." The significance of the relation of food production to population control is readily understood; it is evident that we may multiply ourselves into population extinction by starvation. But we are told, too, that we may also multiply ourselves into intellectual extinction so that we should no longer be uniquely human. Our concern is, therefore, not just with the survival of man's body but his intellect as well. This is an intriguing concept with respect to population control.

It is essential that birth rates be cut radically and promptly. But how? It is the how that Dr. Rock describes, principally in terms of the recommendations of the United Nations Mission in India, a country where each year the population increases by more than ten million. The methods of control that Dr. Rock discusses are: raising the age of marriage; sterilization of either husband or wife; the condom; the pill; and the intra-uterine device.

With all of these methods combined, it is estimated that the growth rate in India could be stopped in ten years; in a decade there would be no more births there than deaths. This, of course, assumes much, including a knowledge of what the death rate would be ten years hence. It also assumes that many of the problems related to motivation such as ignorance, illiteracy, adequate medical and paramedical personnel, superstition and cultural background, somehow can all be resolved. This is quite obviously a considerable assumption.

The inevitable conclusion arises that we shall need better methods of control, and these methods will include more than merely better pills or better techniques of contraception. The answer to a more satisfactory pill may prove to be easier than the answer to the over-all problem of population control. We may develop a practical pill but not the motivation to use it or the means or the will to deliver it or apply it.

Pertinent to the types of pills currently in use, we hear much of their possible serious side effects. Dr. Lasagna, in particular, suggested that the possible harmful side effects of the pill weigh heavily against its benefits. To be sure we must bear these considerations in mind. But they must be weighed against the possible harm of not using the pill. For example, how many deaths could reasonably be attributed to the pill as compared to the approximately ten thousand deaths from illegal abortions that we have been told occurred in this country last year. Also, how much illness can be attributed to the pill in comparison to that endured by the roughly 300,000 women who annually end up in hospitals for the treatment of hemorrhage, infection, or other complications of illegal surgery.

The problem of criminal abortion inescapably leads to the topic of legalized abortions. Any discussion of population control must consider the role of legalized abortions. To consider this matter is not to condone it. And to condemn it is not to ignore it. Dr. Rock personally regards abortion as a preventable problem. The larger problem of birth control, however, is clearly extremely complex. Most masterfully he has given us a graceful, rounded, and authoritative discussion of this difficult, sensitive, and vastly significant topic.

Linked with birth control is the opposite force of the death rate. More people now live longer than ever before in history. In no small measure this phenomenon is due to the discovery and development of the twentieth century's great weapon against infection, the antibiotics.

This story, as unfolded by Dr. Weinstein, began with the rumblings that preceded the chance discovery of penicillin by Fleming; it then passed through a dormant period to the flowering of the antibiotic era, when we saw the massive cooperative effort on the part of universities, industry, and government. The saga, as Dr. Weinstein told it, then proceeded through the conquest of disease after disease with the spectacular saving of lives, the relief of suffering, and the prevention of illness. These achievements made themselves felt on the battlefield as well.

Next we learned something about the mechanisms by which the cure of infection is accomplished.

But we also were warned of the dark side of what Dr. Weinstein calls the antibiotic coin. For antibiotics may lose their effectiveness, and as we found out, they do have great capacity for harm. They are also at times overused and otherwise improperly prescribed.

But over-all, as he so well noted, antibiotic treatment is easily the greatest therapeutic achievement of this century. The evolution of this treatment points up many major themes in the emergence of any new drug. There is the almost frightening importance of chance observation as well as the disturbing thought that the unraveling that should follow an original glimpse into a potential therapeutic miracle might never take place. It was a fortunate combination of circumstances—eleven years after Fleming's observations—that led to the practical use of penicillin. Had it not been for the Oxford group of Florey, Chain, and Abraham, who knows? Fleming's observations might still be buried in the medical literature waiting to be accidentally discovered. This is not an isolated example of the delay that may occur in moving from observations of great potential value to their practical application. Other instances that quickly come to mind are catheterization of the heart and the sulfa drugs. How many more reports are concealed in scientific data and journals waiting to be exploited for man's benefit?

Then there is in the glorious story of antibiotics, in addition to the miracle of chance discovery, the shining example of the development of a new drug through well-planned and what Dr. Lasagna called rigorous experimentation. I refer to Dr. Selman Waksman and the discovery of streptomycin.

Dr. Weinstein also depicted the important place of industry in the development of drugs; the need for controls by government; the necessity of caution by physicians and restraint by patients; the place of drugs in preventive medicine and public health; the recently recognized problems of drug resistance and the older ones of drug reactions; and the need for suppressing the exuberance that naturally attends the introduction of a new drug and, especially, a useful one.

There is hardly a principle in the evolution of new drugs that is not seen in greatly magnified form in the engrossing antibiotic story. Dr. Weinstein has touched upon them all, the good and the bad, the admirable and the somber, the exciting and the cheerless. But above all, he has given us a sense of the feeling that comes from the bright glow of a wondrous discovery, in particular a discovery that is aimed solely at human well-being.

To evaluate adequately the safety of drugs, however, it has become abundantly clear that testing must include not only effects on the patient under treatment but also upon the living system even before birth. Moreover, this aspect of drug safety— certainty that medicines are in no way harmful to the fragile embryo or fetus—has led to a new focus of attention on the most intimate relationship in life, the symbiosis of pregnancy.

It appears that we shall have to look anew at the extent to which the placenta serves as a barrier to possible harmful substances. Dr. Gellis not only made clear the need for identification of these substances and a reappraisal of the placenta's barrier role, but he has given an informative account of what is happening to enlarge our understanding of the problem. He cites a number of specific examples of harmful substances, which gain access to the circulation of the fetus, beginning with the "thalidomide disaster." It was thalidomide that spurred a large-scale exploration of the relatively new science of teratology, the study of malformations. We learn that the highest risk of induced malformations in the fetus is during the first weeks of pregnancy, when organs are in the process of formation.

Dr. Gellis tells us that about 2 per cent of all living newborn infants have abnormalities recognizable at birth and by one year of age an additional 1 to 2 per cent are shown to have abnormalities that existed but were not detected at delivery. In 90 per cent of these instances the cause of the abnormality is still unknown. We are told that the effects of many drugs that are widely used separately and in combinations are now being re-examined in this regard. The first one to be definitely associated with the induction of abnormalities in the fetus was the anticancer agent, aminopterin, in 1952. The list of other agents that may be harmful during the early development of the unborn child is long and the effects are varied. This list includes: hormones (progesterone, cortisone, thyroid); narcotics; antibiotics; sulfonamides; and common drugs such as barbiturates, antihistamines, antidepressants, aspirin and other salicylates, phenacetin, and vitamins.

Special mention is made by Dr. Gellis of the possible harmful consequences of X-rays, and he warns that X-ray studies should not be conducted in women during the early period of pregnancy unless they are absolutely necessary. In fact, such a warning would apply as well to almost any drug until there is much more knowledge than we now have of what the possible harmful effects of such a drug might be.

Dr. Gellis has given us information of great public significance, and he has brought to bear on it a critique that allows an intelligent evaluation of the present state of our knowledge of the importance of drugs to the unborn child. We have in his discussion an example of the extreme difficulties that one encounters in grasping the full significance of a new area of drug study. The need at this time for caution is therefore obvious and clear.

Another world of drug use, perhaps the one with the greatest potential for the future, lies within the dark sphere of mental illness. An account of the present state of drug therapy in patients with mental illness reminds us that the drug approach is quite new, is still exploratory, and is most promising. These are, perhaps, the three key summary words, *new, exploratory,* and *promising.*

It would appear that drugs for mental illness have not yet reached such a level of effectiveness that we can abandon psychotherapy in one form or another. But we may still hope—as Freud himself hoped some thirty years ago—that drugs will make much of the time-consuming and often somewhat unsatisfactory psychotherapy less necessary. In this respect there is remarkable pertinence in a quote from a small book written by Freud shortly before he died. It was indeed the last of his writings, an effort directed to the general public and entitled *An Outline of Psychoanalysis.*

It is true that we do not always succeed in winning, but at least we can usually see why it is that we have not won. Those who have been following our discussion only out of therapeutic interest will perhaps turn away in contempt after this admission. But we are here concerned with therapy only in so far as it works by psychological methods; and for the time being we have no other. The future may teach us how to exercise a direct influence, by means of particular chemical substances, upon . . . the apparatus of the mind. It may be that there are other undreamed-of possibilities of therapy. But for the moment we have nothing better at our disposal than the technique of psychoanalysis, and for that reason, in spite of its limitations, it is not to be despised.

We are now in that future to which Freud referred: "the future that will teach us how to exercise a direct influence [on the apparatus of the mind] by means of particular chemical substance." Dr. Cole has been talking about the advances that are being made toward finding those "particular chemical substances" that would beneficially affect the behavior of the mind.

As Dr. Cole indicated, we now are witnessing the early unfolding of an approach that may ultimately contribute as much to man's happiness as anything that science can offer, namely the eradication of mental illness.

Freud's contribution came through the penetrating application of sheer intellectual power to an understanding of the psychological functioning of the mind. Now perhaps some intellectual power, applied at the laboratory bench, plus perhaps a "little bit o' luck" will enable us to learn something about the biological behavior of the mind, and what we may do to alter it favorably as the occasion demands.

This is the area that Dr. Cole has opened for thoughtful consideration. There is much that is fascinating in what he has told and there is much that lies just out of reach. Of his presentation, therefore, it must be said that it is in effect the first installment of a story that is "to be continued." For there will surely be many more chapters in the years to come.

The drug story that the public as well as the medical profession would like most to read, however, is one that would carry happy endings in cases of cancer. Of great interest in this regard is the increasing role being assigned in the grim drama of cancer to the patient's own system of defenses.

The keynote of Dr. Friedkin's report has been cautious optimism and a plea for a predominantly rational, rather than a grossly empirical, approach to cancer therapy. This will still leave room for the chance observation, one that could even come from a totally unrelated field. We cannot plan to have someone stumble upon a vital observation, but if the history of drugs teaches anything, it teaches that we should not be surprised by some such happy accident. It would be fine if we could somehow go about multiplying the chances of a spectacular chance observation, that is, multiply the possibilities of someone stumbling onto a cancer cure. But this seems somewhat illusory, although to be sure we might move toward such a goal by creating more "prepared minds," *i.e.,* minds prepared to take suitable advantage of a chance observation.

What may not be illusory, however, is the possibility of an approach through a better understanding of inborn control mechanisms. It is because of these control mechanisms that many of us will not succumb to the effects of abnormal cell growth. Clinicians speak of "self-limited" diseases. And fortunately most diseases are self-limited. If they weren't, few if any of us would ever reach adulthood. Why is a disease self-limited? It is because nature has provided certain mechanisms for the control of a given abnormal process. In the case of infections these are called "immune mechanisms." In the case of cancer there must also be some defense mechanisms. Otherwise, how can one account for the fact that where two persons appear to have the same cancer, and to the same extent, one rapidly succumbs while the other goes on living normally.

Dr. Friedkin noted that only 12 per cent of patients with cancer of the stomach survive for five years if the cancer is treated late and after it has spread regionally. Only 5 per cent of patients with lung cancer survive under the same circumstances. What are the factors—the so-called host factors—that the 5 per cent of patients who survived the lung cancer had, and evidently the 95 per cent who succumbed did not have?

How do we account for the fact that a certain type of white-blood-cell proliferation will in one person be self-limited and be called infectious mononucleosis, whereas in another person a proliferation of similar cells will be self-perpetuating and be called leukemia?

Nature appears to provide some of us with protective host factors, in effect a still deeply concealed arsenal of weapons with which to fight malignant cell growth. It remains for the biochemist, the pharmacologist, and the clinician to learn what these weapons are and how to apply them to eliminate one of man's greatest scourges—cancer.

The largest area of medical concern is coming to be that of the degenerative diseases. And the most important of the degenerative diseases are those due to atherosclerosis or "hardening of the arteries." The dramatic evidences of such arterial change are heart attacks and strokes. But atherosclerosis also produces insidious damage to vital organs; for example, involvement of the arteries supplying blood to the brain may cause mental deterioration.

As more people live to an older age, more people are subjected to the disability and death that accompany atherosclerosis. It is little wonder, therefore, that in the discussion of heart attacks and strokes we are told that "cardiovascular disease is easily the greatest medical problem facing America today." We are also told, understandably, that if we are to prolong useful life, we shall have to prevent or cure, or at least slow the atherosclerotic process. Obviously the best approach is prevention.

In order to prevent heart attacks and strokes we need to know what causes atherosclerosis. While we really don't know its cause, we believe we do know what appears to favor its development. That is, we know what factors make a person more prone to heart attacks and strokes. Among these the ones that are subject to modification by drugs are high blood pressure and high blood fats (as measured usually by cholesterol levels). Because the drug nicotine is probably responsible for the harmful effects of cigarettes on the arteries, cigarette smoking is also discussed. The essence of the discussion on cigarette smoking is contained in the following statement:

> When we realize that up to two-thirds of all heart deaths due to coronary artery disease in cigarette smokers may be prevented by the simple expedient of stopping cigarette smoking, we begin to comprehend the magnitude of the preventive possibilities. There is probably no area in medicine today in which preventive measures have more to offer.

We now have drugs that will lower blood pressure and blood fats. We shall, therefore, in a few years be able to answer the question as to whether the correction of elevated levels of blood pressure and blood fats will delay the appearance of heart attacks and strokes.

The plethora of drugs available today not only makes for difficult choices in determining proper use, but presages real trouble when the dispensing hand is too generous, albeit well-intentioned. Too many drugs now are recognized to be inducers of disease states.

This topic, explored by Dr. Moser, is relatively new to medicine and completely new as a subject of considerable magnitude. It concerns a large and growing segment of illnesses to which attention is being appropriately and increasingly directed. Its importance becomes evident in light of one recent study identifying as many as 13 per cent of all hospital deaths as seemingly caused by drugs intended to save lives.

In his lively and fascinating review of this new field, Dr. Moser has introduced his descriptive term, "diseases of medical progress." This theme provided a topic in a talk given by one of our

(Tufts) Medical School professors to the graduating class last year. In viewing the full sweep of medical progress in his lifetime, he concluded that we had finally reached the point where all illnesses could be put into three categories: those cured by antibiotics, those helped by cortisone, and those caused by antibiotics and cortisone.

Obviously this was said in jest. But as is so often the case in such witticisms, there is more than a grain of truth in the remark. Thus we have learned specifically about the illnesses that are produced by cortisone. Dr. Moser selected the corticosteroids as a prototype for his discussion. This was a happy choice. For here we have an extremely useful drug; there can be no question of its efficacy. And it also is a drug that was widely hailed and enthusiastically prescribed for some time before many of its faults began to be evident. Dr. Moser portrayed vividly the gradual recognition of more and more harmful side effects.

But we must guard against the dangers of distortion when our attention is focused on just the ill effects of useful drugs. We must remember that generally we are dealing with rare effects. And these instances are thrown into sharp relief for the purpose of emphasizing a point. Dr. Moser properly emphasized that the real benefits of the corticosteroids so outweigh the occasional harm as to leave no doubt about their over-all value.

It's as though one were given a vivid description of the scene of an airplane wreck in which there are mangled bodies and scattered remnants of the plane; and then told that this is what may happen if one flies. The risk of such an experience, dreadful though it is, is so slight that we ignore it. We make such calcuations, in effect, whenever we take a drug of any sort. For that matter, the same is true of surgery. We ask ourselves if the benefits of a particular operation outweigh the risk. When the answer is *yes,* we accept the odds. Incidentally, as Dr. Moser makes clear in his book, *Diseases of Medical Progress,* such diseases not only result from drugs but may be surgically induced as well. To summarize some of his points:

A flood of new drugs has come at a time in the progress of medicine when, fortunately, it is possible to find out a great deal about their effects, good and bad; effects on normal as well as diseased tissue.

There are certain inherited variants of tissue behavior revealed only by the effects of drugs; a phenomenon that has given rise to a new field in medicine known as "pharmacogenetics."

There are important residual and late consequences of drugs and important aspects of the interaction of drugs, the effect of one drug acting upon another.

New modes of drug administration—what Dr. Moser calls "these unprecedented therapeutic intrusions"—have been graphically emphasized.

But fresh help is coming to the rescue of the unfortunate physician today, who is overwhelmed by the avalanche of new drugs. The help is to be supplied by the American Medical Association's Council on Drugs and by the Federal Drug Administration. These agencies, Dr. Moser acknowledges, by disseminating timely, trustworthy, and unbiased data, will do much to keep physicians suitably informed of the hazards that lurk in their prescription pads.

Behind the appearance of every new drug lie batteries of tests, including trial doses given humans. When the number of new drugs is multiplied by the number of tests, the enormity of experimental drug testing becomes apparent. And the ethical questions raised by the extent, however necessary, of such testing are formidable and unavoidable.

Dr. Chalmers underscored the fact that science and ethics are wholly compatible. Indeed, the scientific approach to human drug trials may be the more ethical approach, since it involves carefully gathered knowledge, controlled use, and expertly studied responses. What we strive for is the scientific method applied under the guidance of the Golden Rule, in either its negative or positive form. In its negative form it is: Do not unto others as you would not have them do unto you. That much should be unequivocal. In its positive version—Do unto others as you would have them do unto you—it should be applied with the intelligence and protection of science; for the mind and the heart together can be better than either alone. That, in fact, is the basis of the practice of medicine itself.

The scientific testing of the effects of drugs on human subjects is a comparatively new field and one that is still evolving. The medical profession is developing an awareness of the significance and importance of random assignment of cases, proper controls, double-blind testing, placebos, and statistical validity. Physicians are also struggling with the meaning of informed consent and just how to protect those who volunteer for testing.

With grace and clarity Dr. Chalmers has described the four phases through which the process of human drug-testing moves, namely: the initial trial in volunteers; the initial trial in patients; the controlled clinical trial; and finally the field trials. This is a reasonable and logical pathway which steers between a degree of caution, which would make it almost impossible to introduce new drugs, and one of carelessness, which would be dangerous to the public welfare.

He properly pointed out what is often forgotten: Doctors are daily "testing" drugs in their practice. This they frequently do in situations where the diagnosis is not clear and at times they do it in an effort to establish a diagnosis by a therapeutic response. Thus, in the differential diagnosis of gout and rheumatoid arthritis, for example, a good response to colchicine will suggest that the correct diagnosis is gout because the discomfort of gout usually clears with colchicine, while that of rheumatoid arthritis does not.

The individual physician working with the individual patient must test drugs on the basis of a happy blend of conscience, knowledge, experience, and care. In effect, Dr. Chalmers has reminded us that this same combination applies in the whole sweep of human drug trials, a combination of the old and the new, the old Golden Rule and the new scientific method.

It is assumed that the good physician must be well informed. But he must also be thoughtful, careful, and kind. These qualities that we prize so highly in the practicing physician are also the qualities that enable the science and the ethics of human drug testing to coexist so harmoniously, congenially, and profitably for mankind.

To appreciate how far the practice of medicine has come in the development of drugs occasionally requires a backward glance. And it adds perspective to look outward at the support given by kindred contributors in sciences that followed different but parallel roads.

Dr. Keefer has done that. He has contrasted for us the status of drugs today and in Osler's time during the latter part of the nineteenth century, and that contrast is striking. In that bygone era Dr. Oliver Wendell Holmes, the father of the Justice, said something to the effect that if, with a few exceptions such as opium and anesthetics, all of the drugs in the pharmacopoeia of his day were dumped into the ocean, it would be good for mankind but bad for the fish. Were Dr. Holmes living today, however, he would likely be telling his medical students of the millions of lives that have been spared and of the untold suffering that has been eliminated through the proper use of the drugs in our modern pharmacopoeia.

Dr. Keefer has given us a factual picture based on first-hand knowledge. He has spoken chiefly of the contributions of industry, and there is a need for this emphasis, for in recent years we have been flooded with criticism of the pharmaceutical industry. Surely the industry has its faults. It is easy to give a biased portrayal of the virtues or the faults as the case may be. You will recall the story of the historian who wrote what he called an unbiased account of the Civil War from the point of view of a Southerner. When such a book is written, then someone else must write a similarly so-called unbiased account from a Northerner's point of view. What we need, it seems, is a balance of biases.

Seriously we should be made aware of our indebtedness to the drug industry, and no one is more familiar with the true nature of that indebtedness than Dr. Keefer. Nor is anyone better qualified to give us the perspective that places the drug industry in its proper position in the over-all picture, a picture that also contains university, research institute, government, physician, and patient.

Dr. Keefer has spelled out the respective roles of these participants. All have their particular problems, their distinctive concerns, and their special immediate motivations. But also, all have overlapping concerns and interests. It is the reconciling of all of these that requires what Dr. Keefer calls "hearty and harmonious collaboration." Out of this collaboration will come the fullest measure of the contributions drugs can make to man's health and happiness.

From long personal experience Dr. Keefer knows what the collaborative effort for which he pleads can mean. It was with such cooperation on the part of government, science, and industry, and under the guidance of Dr. Keefer, that the history of drugs had its finest hour: the development, production, and distribution of penicillin.

It is helpful to think of medicine as a continuum that extends from the molecule at one extreme to society at the other. In the center is man. And it is man who is the concern of the physician. At one end the concern is principally that of the molecular biologist; at the other, of the social scientist. At one end man is viewed in terms of a molecule and at the other, as a statistic. The drug industry must concern itself with the full progression from molecular biology to social science. And Dr. Keefer has given a graphic account of what this broad involvement on the part of the pharmaceutical industry means ultimately to the person who takes a drug.

He has underscored the important issues that will determine what the future holds for the development of new drugs and the improvement of old ones. These issues, namely, professionalism, economic philosophy, and national research policy are vitally important. They need to be dispassionately debated, they demand clarification, and we must have sound and wise decisions made with respect to the questions they raise if the health of our society is to be what it can and should be. As the issues are clarified, and as wise decisions are made, we shall in all likelihood find ourselves turning to the drug industry, which alone is in a position to deliver the goods.

How much of this will come to pass depends today to an increasing degree on the controls imposed on drug development, from discovery right across the system through production and distribution. As with all other aspects of drugs, control is tantalizingly complex.

Dr. Goddard has given us a historical background that is most helpful in placing his efforts and those of the entire Food and Drug Administration in perspective. The agency began with the control of harmful drugs, a function obviously in the public interest. But the degree of harmfulness and indeed the definition of harmful raises questions that are not easily answered.

The newer government regulations now require judgments as to drug effectiveness. In a sense this is reasonable, for in order to establish a relationship between harm and benefit one must measure effectiveness. But neither harmful nor beneficial effects are readily determined. For example, after twenty years we are still finding hitherto unknown harmful side effects of some of the antibiotics. Surely we cannot wait twenty years to be told whether a drug is too toxic to be given a seal of approval. Also after twenty years there still is considerable controversy as to whether anticlotting drugs are helpful in treating heart attacks. Again, we can't wait twenty years to be told whether a drug is efficacious.

The basic problem confronting the FDA in its necessary efforts to protect the public is that so many of the decisions they must make deal with questions that fall in a large gray area where the proper answer is extremely difficult to ascertain.

The side effects may not just be long in making themselves evident; they also may be difficult to interpret. Thus, the person who becomes drowsy after taking an antihistamine tablet and as a result is killed in an automobile accident, in effect has had a fatal reaction to an antihistamine. The direct effect is drowsiness, but the indirect effect is death.

Or a person who commits suicide as a result of a depression induced by a drug that lowers blood pressure (Reserpine) has experienced a fatal complication of an efficacious and apparently safe drug. The direct effect was depression; the indirect one, death.

Who is to judge the efficacy of drugs, when the benefits may not be immediate or unequivocal? The late Sir Thomas Lewis of London, one of the greatest of modern cardiologists, was convinced in 1930 that digitalis, then in use for some 150 years, was worthless in patients with heart failure when the heart rhythm was regular. On the other hand the late Henry Christian, a professor at Harvard and one of this country's most distinguished clinicians and teachers, was convinced (also about 1930) that digitalis was beneficial in patients with simple elevation of blood pressure even without evidence of heart disease. It now is clear that Lewis and Christian were both wrong. Yet no one in the first half of this century spoke with greater authority than they.

To be sure we have more precise methods today for measuring drug efficacy in humans, but there still remains an area for individual judgment. Is that to be forsaken, and with what results?

A drug may be found to be relatively ineffective as an antihistamine or as a muscle relaxant and hence not approved for use. Were this to happen today we might never have known about Thorazine and Meprobamate, and the progress of the drug treatment of mental illness would have been seriously hampered. We must leave room for serendipity.

Practicing physicians need to learn about drug actions, good and bad. Who is to take the responsibility for developing an educational program that will provide this essential information? Is this responsibility to be left to the individual physician, his medical school, his medical society, medical journals, the government, or drug houses? Here is an area ideally suited to a well-organized and adequately subsidized collaborative effort.

With the completion of the series one is struck anew by the sweep and span of the subject: the depth of each aspect—the drugs, the diseases for which they are given, and those that they may cause; the patient for whom they are prescribed and the society they affect.

Much has truly changed since eighteenth century practices prompted Voltaire to protest bitterly: "Doctors pour in drugs about which they know little to treat diseases of which they know less in human beings of whom they know nothing."

Yet, if these reflections have shown anything, it is that the wonder of drugs, not to mention the full knowledge of man and his role in society, are matters still but dimly perceived.

The hope has been expressed that in the year 2000 there might be a series of Lowell Lectures on "The Un-Medicated Society." This may indeed by a vain hope. Short of that, however, perhaps we may look forward to a series not too many years hence entitled "The Properly Medicated Society."

General Reading References

Edward Weeks, *The Lowells and Their Institute,* Boston, Atlantic-Little, Brown and Company, 1966.

Paul Talalay, Ed., *Drugs in Our Society,* Baltimore, Johns Hopkins University Press, 1964.

Louis Lasagna, M.D., *The Doctor's Dilemmas,* New York, Harpers Bros., 1962; paperback by Collier Books, 1963.

S. Cohen, *The Beyond Within: The LSD Story* New York, Athenaeum Publishers, 1964.

Donald Lauria, M.D., *Nightmare Drugs,* New York, Pocket Books Inc., 1964.

I. Chein, D.L. Gerard, R.S. Lee, and E. Rosenfeld, *The Road to H,* New York, Basic Books Inc., 1964.

William and Paul Paddock, *Famine in 1975,* Boston, Little, Brown and Company, 1967.

John Rock, M.D., *The Time Has Come—A Catholic Doctor's Proposals to End the Battle Over Birth Control,* New York, Alfred A. Knopf, Inc., 1963.

Gregory Pincus, *Control of Fertility,* New York, Academic Press, Inc., 1965.

Howard W. Haggard, M.D., *Devils, Drugs and Doctors,* New York, Harpers & Bros., Blue Ribbon Books, 1929.

Harvey Graham (Isaac Flack) *Eternal Eve,* London, Hutchinson, 1960.

F. O. Kelsey, *Action of Drugs on the Embryo: Drug-Induced Dis-*

eases, eds., L. Meyler and H. M. Peck, International Congress Series, No. 85. Excerpta Medica Foundation, July 1965.

Max Rinkel, M.D., Ed., *Biological Treatment of Mental Illness,* Copyright, the Manfred Sakel Foundation; New York, L.C. Page & Co., 1966.

R. Goldstein, *One in Seven: Drugs on Campus,* New York, Walker & Co., 1966.

Pat McGrady, *The Savage Cell—A Report on Cancer and Cancer Research,* New York, Basic Books, Inc., 1964.

Smoking and Health, Report of the Advisory Committee to the Surgeon General of the Public Health Service, U.S. Dept. of Health, Education and Welfare, 1964, Publication No. 1103.

Arthur Selzer, M.D., *The Heart: Its Function in Health and Disease,* Berkeley and Los Angeles, University of California Press, 1966.

Alton Blakeslee, Jr., and Jeremiah Stamler, M.D., *Your Heart Has Nine Lives: Nine Steps to Heart Health,* Englewood, New Jersey, Prentice-Hall, Inc., 1963.

Morton Mintz, *Therapeutic Nightmare,* Boston, Houghton Mifflin Company; Cambridge, Massachusetts, The Riverside Press, 1965.

Herman Miles Somers and Anne Ramsey Somers, *Doctors, Patients and Health Insurance,* Washington, D.C., The Brookings Institute, 1961.

Rachel Carson, *Silent Spring,* Boston, Houghton Mifflin Company, 1962.

Clinical Investigation in Medicine: Legal, Ethical and Moral Aspects, Edited by Law-Medicine Research Institute, Boston University, 1963.

A National Program to Conquer Heart Disease, Cancer and Stroke, The President's Commission on Heart Disease, Cancer and Stroke, Document Number 0-763-310, Washington, D.C., U.S. Government Printing Office, February 1965.

Index

[267]

DATE DUE